The Educational Resource Library asks that you please return your library materials when you are done with them. If they have been helpful to you, they will help another. If you would like to purchase this title, please contact the librarian and she can assist you with your purchase. This Library copy is not for sale.

MAYO CLINIC

The
Menopause
Solution

Published by Time Inc. Books
225 Liberty Street, New York, NY 10281

© 2016 Mayo Foundation for Medical Education and Research (MFMER)

ISBN-10: 0-8487-4675-9
ISBN-13: 978-0-8487-4675-9

Library of Congress Control Number: 2016934092

10 9 8 7 6 5 4 3 2 1

Mayo Clinic The Menopause Solution is intended to supplement the advice of your personal physician, whom you should consult regarding individual medical conditions. The information in the book is general and is offered with no guarantees on the part of the author or publisher. The author and publisher disclaim all liability in connection with the use of this book. We do not endorse any company or product. MAYO, MAYO CLINIC and the Mayo triple-shield logo are marks of Mayo Foundation for Medical Education and Research.

For bulk sales to employers, member groups and health-related companies, contact Mayo Clinic, 200 First St. SW, Rochester, MN 55905, call 800-430-9699, or send an email to *SpecialSales MayoBooks@Mayo.edu.*

Printed in the United States of America

Big rocks analogy, pages 312-313, is provided with permission by Franklin Covey Co.

Sections on gratitude and mindfulness, Chapters 18 and 19, are based on content from *The Mayo Clinic Guide to Stress-Free Living,* by Amit Sood, © 2013. Reprinted by permission of Da Capo Lifelong Books, a member of The Perseus Books Group.

PHOTO CREDITS

There is no correlation between the individuals portrayed and the conditions or subjects discussed.

PAGE: V/CREDIT: © MAYO FOUNDATION FOR MEDICAL EDUCATION AND RESEARCH (MFMER) – NAME: 56972323.PSD/PAGE 34/CREDIT: © THINKSTOCK – NAME: 505567555.JPG/PAGE 68/CREDIT: © THINKSTOCK – NAME: 00171411-001.PSD/PAGE 81/CREDIT: © THINKSTOCK – NAME: 56162812_14.PSD/PAGE 90/CREDIT: © GETTY IMAGES – NAME: 180412768.PSD/PAGE 93/CREDIT: © THINKSTOCK – NAME: 106569410.JPG/PAGE 101/CREDIT: © THINKSTOCK – NAME: 180412764.JPG.PSD/PAGE 107/CREDIT: © THINKSTOCK – NAME: 78739800.PSD/PAGE 117/CREDIT: © THINKSTOCK – NAME: BLDJP03232004_69.PSD/PAGE 119/CREDIT: © THINKSTOCK – NAME: 114333375.JPG/PAGE 131/CREDIT: © THINKSTOCK – NAME: 78023425.PSD/PAGE 157/CREDIT: © THINKSTOCK – NAME: 469767232.PSD/PAGE 162/CREDIT: © THINKSTOCK – NAME: SKD284305SDC_22.PSD/PAGE 178/CREDIT: © GETTY IMAGES – NAME: 200258063-001.PSD/PAGE 184/CREDIT: © THINKSTOCK – NAME: 463394757.PSD/PAGE 211/CREDIT: © THINKSTOCK – NAME: 67078.PSD/PAGE 224/CREDIT: © GETTY IMAGES – NAME: 78752095.PSD/PAGE 228/CREDIT: © THINKSTOCK – NAME: 67114.PSD/PAGE 244/CREDIT: © GETTY IMAGES – NAME: 78461846.PSD/PAGE 246/CREDIT: © THINKSTOCK – NAME: 100577216.PSD/PAGE 257/CREDIT: © THINKSTOCK – NAME: 57448489.PSD/PAGE 261/CREDIT: © THINKSTOCK – NAME: 110070.PSD/PAGE 263/CREDIT: © GETTY IMAGES – NAME: 469077198.PSD/PAGE 269/CREDIT: © THINKSTOCK – NAME: 177817016.PSD/PAGE 291/CREDIT: © THINKSTOCK – NAME: 486487577.JPG/PAGE 291/CREDIT: © THINKSTOCK – NAME: 489245560.PSD/PAGE 296/CREDIT: © THINKSTOCK – NAME: 84523071.PSD/PAGE 305/CREDIT: © THINKSTOCK – NAME: 461261395.PSD/PAGE 308/CREDIT: © THINKSTOCK – NAME: 464821723.PSD/PAGE 312/CREDIT: © THINKSTOCK – NAME: 461272765.JPG/PAGE 319/CREDIT: © THINKSTOCK – NAME: DV-2051009VR2.PSD/PAGE 323/CREDIT: © GETTY IMAGES

MAYO CLINIC

Medical Editor
Stephanie S. Faubion, M.D.

Managing Editor
Jennifer L. Jacobson

Contributors
Samantha A. Alley
Rachel A. H. Bartony
Alicia C. Bartz
Bart L. Clarke, M.D.
Paru S. David, M.D.
Julia A. Files, M.D.
Amy L. Frye
Karthik Ghosh, M.D.
Karen Grothe, Ph.D., L.P.
Donald D. Hensrud, M.D., M.P.H.
Ekta Kapoor, M.B.B.S.
Kurt A. Kennel, M.D.
Juliana (Jewel) M. Kling, M.D., M.P.H.
Jennifer Haugen Koski
Carol L. Kuhle, D.O.
Edward R. Laskowski, M.D.
Melissa C. Lipford, M.D.
Rekha Mankad, M.D.
Anita P. Mayer, M.D.
Denise M. Millstine, M.D.
Sharon L. Mulvagh, M.D.
Walter A. Rocca, M.D.
Jordan Rullo, Ph.D., L.P.
Nicole P. Sandhu, M.D., Ph.D.
Richa Sood, M.D.
Jacqueline M. Thielen, M.D.
Dawn B. Underwood, P.T., D.P.T.
Suneela Vegunta, M.D.
Karen R. Wallevand
Laura Hamilton Waxman

Editorial Director
Paula M. Marlow Limbeck

Project Manager
Christopher C. Frye

Illustrators and Photographers
Joseph M. Kane
James Postier

Research Librarians
Anthony J. Cook
Deirdre A. Herman
Erika A. Riggin

Proofreaders
Miranda M. Attlesey
Alison K. Baker
Julie M. Maas

Indexer
Steve Rath

Administrative Assistant
Beverly J. Steele
Terri L. Zanto Strausbauch

TIME INC. BOOKS

Editor
Meredith L. Butcher

Senior Manager, Business Development and Partnerships
Nina Reed

Project Editor
Lacie Pinyan

Art Director
Christopher Rhoads

Assistant Production Manager
Diane Rose Keener

Design Fellow
Olivia Pierce

Cover design by Christopher Rhoads

PREFACE

The idea for this book has developed over the last few years and is based on my experiences working with women going through the menopausal transition. In my practice, I've been struck by the lack of unbiased, reliable information available to women about menopause and its treatment. Women often have a talk in elementary school about their menstrual cycles and some limited sex education, and they may have a review about what's happening to their bodies when they have a baby, but there's no class to prepare for what happens to their bodies at midlife! Not infrequently, I see women who travel across the country to find an explanation for their bothersome and mysterious symptoms, only to find out that what they are experiencing is, indeed, a normal process.

Knowledge is powerful. Simply understanding what's happening, and that it's a natural part of life, can be reassuring. Although there's still much to learn about menopause, including what exactly causes a hot flash, more is being understood every day. One thing is very clear, however — there isn't a single solution for the menopausal symptoms that women experience. Today, more than ever, treatments for menopause are personalized and individualized, based on women's symptoms, medical and family history, and personal values and preferences.

With hormone therapy, for example, one size does not fit all. Some women will never need hormone therapy. They might not have bothersome hot flashes or night sweats or difficulty with sleeping, concentrating or mood issues — some never have a single hot flash. But most women do have some symptoms that accompany this transition phase. And when the symptoms are troublesome enough to consider hormone therapy, the regimen, dose and route of administration may vary depending on her specific circumstances.

For some women, menopause may not occur at the normal time, but may come early — whether it's related to removal of the ovaries, treatment of cancer or due to early loss of ovarian function for unclear reasons. For these women, symptoms may be especially severe, and unless there's a clear reason to avoid it, treatment with hormone therapy is particularly important to prevent the long-term health consequences of losing estrogen too soon.

There also are women who may have very bothersome menopausal symptoms, but are either unable or choose not to take hormone therapy. For these women, there are effective nonhormonal options for managing symptoms that this book will share.

It's becoming clear that menopausal symptoms aren't as limited
in duration as was previously
thought. In fact, it's now understood that hot flashes and night
sweats last, on average, for more
than seven years. This is why it's
important to find a solution that
works for you, as the symptoms
may be around for a while! Even
more bothersome than hot flashes
and night sweats can be some of
the other signs and symptoms
related to menopause, including
weight gain, fatigue, sleep disturbances, mood changes and sexual
function changes. Understanding

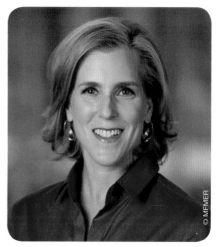

Stephanie S. Faubion, M.D.
Medical editor

what is happening to your body and what you can do about it is key. I
often tell my patients, "The rules of your body have changed and no one
told you." That's why this book was written: To tell you what's happening
to you and what you can do about it.

This book was inspired by the women with hormonal and sexual health
concerns I see every day in the Women's Health Clinic at Mayo Clinic in
Rochester, Minnesota and by my colleagues who have devoted their
clinical and research careers to helping women through this life phase. I
hope you find it informative and useful, regardless of whether you are
perimenopausal and starting to notice some changes, are in menopause
and wondering what to do about your symptoms, or are still premenopausal and just want to learn more about what may be in store.

Thank you to my women's health colleagues at Mayo Clinic's campuses
in Rochester, Minnesota and in Scottsdale, Arizona for sharing their time
and expertise to make this book a comprehensive guide to menopause.

Table of Contents

Getting a head start on menopause

Menopause is a time of significant change. Your body may be acting in ways you aren't used to, and perhaps you're feeling moody, stressed and tired. Just like when you first got your period, the physical changes and feelings you're experiencing may be confusing, overwhelming and even embarrassing. But they don't have to be. By taking a proactive approach and working collaboratively with your health care provider, you can find ways to make this period of your life not only manageable but also actually enjoyable.

This chapter will help you get a handle on the basics of menopause and what you can do to get a head start in managing your symptoms and taking charge of your health. The following five steps will prepare you to face the menopausal transition with confidence.

》 LEARN

Knowledge is power. Learning more about menopause and your body's changes during this transition will help you feel more in control.

The essentials

1 **MENOPAUSE IS NATURAL.** Menopause isn't a disease or condition to be cured — it's a natural and expected phase of every woman's life. Some women will go through this period with relative ease, while others will seek treatment in order to manage their symptoms.

2 **YOU ARE NOT ALONE.** Menopause is an experience shared by women around the world. Over 2 million women a year enter menopause every year — that's 6,000 women a day! As life expectancy has increased, women are now living a third of their lives beyond menopause. There will be over 20 million postmenopausal women in the U.S. by the year 2020. For many women, this can be a rich and fulfilling time of life.

3 **YOUR BODY IS CHANGING.** As you approach menopause, your body is nearing the end of your fertile years. Your ovaries contain fewer eggs, and the levels of the hormones they produce — estrogen and progesterone — start to fluctuate dramatically and eventually decline to very low levels.

4 **SYMPTOMS ARE COMMON.** Because estrogen influences many parts of your body, its declining levels can result in many bothersome symptoms. Symptoms you might experience include irregular periods, hot flashes and night sweats, skin changes, problems sleeping, weight gain, loss of muscle mass, vaginal dryness, changing interest in sex, memory and concentration issues, and mood swings.

5 **THESE CHANGES IMPACT HOW YOU'RE FEELING.** You're going through a significant life transition and it's normal to experience a wide range of emotions. While you may be anxious or sad about the end of your fertile years, this change may feel liberating to some. Your fluctuating hormone levels may be affecting how you feel, and it's likely that your mood is affected by the intensity of your menopausal symptoms.

6 **A WIDE VARIETY OF TREATMENTS ARE AVAILABLE.** There are many options to help manage your symptoms. No option is permanent. Working with your health care provider, you can come up with a plan that's right for you and revisit it as necessary.

7 **YOU ARE UNIQUE!** Your specific experience of menopause may differ greatly from other women's experiences. Your choices about treatment will be shaped by your current health conditions as well as your personal preferences and values. You are in the driver's seat — there's no one-size-fits-all approach to menopause.

What you can do

1 **MONITOR YOUR CYCLES.** If you're still getting your period, make note of the first and last date of bleeding for each cycle, and whether the flow was light, moderate or heavy. Make sure to have a plan for contraception if you want to avoid pregnancy.

2 **LOG YOUR SYMPTOMS.** If you have symptoms, keep a record of when you experience them, their severity and anything that seems to trigger their occurrence. This may help you identify strategies to manage symptoms such as hot flashes. You can find a sample symptom tracker on page 63.

3 **TRACK YOUR MEDICATIONS.** Keep track of any prescription and nonprescription drugs, vitamins, or other supplements you're taking.

4 **STOP SMOKING.** If you smoke, now's a good time to quit. Smoking has many negative health impacts and can also increase your risk of hot flashes.

5 **TALK TO YOUR PROVIDER.** Your health care provider will be your partner as you approach menopause. Sharing the information you've been tracking will be important as you work together to identify options to manage your symptoms.

6 **KEEP LEARNING.** Arming yourself with information will help you better understand your unique situation and allow you to make informed decisions about any treatment you choose to pursue.

)) FOCUS ON FITNESS

Although physical activity is an essential component of a healthy lifestyle at all ages, exercise can be especially important for women during and after the menopausal transition.

The essentials

1 **WEIGHT GAIN TENDS TO HAPPEN WITH AGE.** You may have noticed your waistline expanding or that you've put on a few pounds. Many women gain weight leading up to and after menopause. You may feel as though the rules of your body have changed and your old strategies for weight management are no longer working. You might need to eat less and exercise more just to maintain your current weight. If you have weight to lose, that means even more activity is needed.

2 **MENOPAUSE AFFECTS YOUR BODY COMPOSITION.** The connection between menopause and weight gain is complicated. Though weight gain isn't necessarily caused by menopause, the decline in estrogen does play a role in increasing the fat in your midsection.

3 **TOO MUCH FAT AROUND THE MIDDLE IS HIGH RISK.** Excess weight in general and increased body fat — especially around your abdomen — can have serious implications for your health, increasing your risk of heart disease, type 2 diabetes and high blood pressure as well as breast, uterine (endometrial) and other cancers.

4 **EXERCISE CAN IMPROVE YOUR HEALTH AND POSSIBLY YOUR SYMPTOMS.** Increased physical activity and a healthy diet during menopause can help you maintain and lose weight — reducing the risks of weight-related diseases. Although studies are inconclusive, exercise and weight loss may also help reduce bothersome symptoms such as hot flashes.

5 **EXERCISE CAN BOOST YOUR MOOD.** Even if it doesn't alleviate your physical symptoms, exercise can relieve stress and anxiety, boost your self-esteem, and improve your mental well-being and quality of life.

6 **EXERCISE CAN IMPROVE MEMORY.** Women often complain of feeling forgetful or having a foggy brain during menopause. Regular exercise, including walking, can your improve memory. Regular moderate exercise has been found to lower your risk of memory loss in later years.

What you can do

1 **MAKE A PLAN.** Exercise and a nutritious diet can prevent weight gain, aid in weight loss and help reduce belly fat. But you do have to take initiative in order to reap these benefits. Start by making a fitness plan that includes a variety of activities.

2 **SET REASONABLE GOALS.** How much physical activity is enough? The prevailing recommendations indicate that healthy adult women should get at least 150 minutes of moderate aerobic activity or 75 minutes of vigorous aerobic activity a week — preferably spread throughout the week — and strength training exercises at least twice a week. This may sound like a lot, but break it up into smaller chunks each day — at least 10 minutes a session — so it doesn't seem so daunting.

3 **MOVE MORE.** In addition to carving out dedicated time for exercise, there are many ways you can fit more movement into your day. At work, try walking meetings and fitting in a walk on your lunch break. Consider a standing desk or using a stability ball as a chair. Park further away from the office or store, or get off the bus a few blocks early to get in some extra steps. Walk or jog in place while watching TV, and walk while talking on the phone.

4 **STAY MOTIVATED.** Set yourself up for success by setting realistic, specific and achievable goals. For example, rather than making a general promise to yourself that you'll exercise more, commit to a daily 30-minute walk after dinner. Frequently update your goals, and choose activities you enjoy at an intensity level you can manage.

5 **EAT WELL.** A balanced diet goes hand in hand with physical activity when you're trying to manage your weight. Focus on whole foods — vegetables, fruits, whole grains, lean proteins and healthy fats — and watch portion sizes.

»GET A GOOD NIGHT'S SLEEP

Many women experience poor sleep around the time of menopause. Sleep problems can leave you feeling fatigued and frustrated. Fortunately, there are steps you can take to optimize your bedtime habits and set yourself up for a good night's sleep.

The essentials

1 **SLEEP IS GOOD FOR YOU.** We all know how it feels when we're short on sleep — we can be irritable, moody, stressed, and have a hard time focusing. But poor sleep affects more than just how we feel. Sleep is a critical time during which your brain and body are busy processing the day, resetting your internal clocks, and resting up for the day to come. Lack of sleep can negatively impact your overall functioning and well-being. It can reduce your immune system activity and can also be dangerous, slowing reaction times and resulting in a greater risk of accidents. To function optimally and stay healthy, most adults need between seven to eight hours of sleep a night.

2 **LACK OF SLEEP IS ASSOCIATED WITH WEIGHT GAIN.** At a time when you may already be battling the bulge, this likely comes as unwelcome news. But research suggests that chronic sleep problems can increase your risk of heart disease, diabetes, obesity and high blood pressure — conditions that already tend to be of concern during and after menopause.

3 **SLEEP MAY BE INTERRUPTED FOR MANY REASONS.** Poor sleep around and after menopause isn't associated with just one cause. Night sweats — hot flashes that occur during the night — may have you waking from your sleep drenched in sweat or shivering with cold. A full bladder or incontinence may have you making trips to the bathroom. Stress, depression or anxiety could be keeping you awake at night, or you may just be sleeping poorly without a clear reason why. It's uncertain whether sleep issues around this time are associated with the hormonal changes of menopause, aging or both.

What you can do

1   **STICK TO A SLEEP SCHEDULE.** Go to bed and get up at the same time every day, even on weekends, holidays and days off. Being consistent reinforces your body's internal rhythms and helps promote better sleep at night.

2   **DON'T FORCE IT.** If you can't fall asleep within about 15 minutes, try getting up and doing a relaxing activity such as reading until you are sleepy, then go back to bed. Feeling anxious about falling asleep may make it harder to nod off.

3   **CREATE A BEDTIME ROUTINE.** A consistent routine can give your body the signal it's time for bed. Try relaxing activities such as taking a warm bath, reading or listening to music — preferably with the lights dimmed — to help you wind down. Limit your use of electronic devices, too — the glowing screens inhibit your ability to fall asleep.

4   **GET COMFORTABLE.** Ensure your bedroom is a quiet, dark and relaxing environment, and use it only for sleep and sex. Choose a mattress and pillow you find comfortable.

5   **WATCH WHAT YOU EAT AND DRINK.** Avoid smoking, alcohol and large meals too close to bedtime. And make sure to watch your caffeine intake — caffeine is a stimulant, and recent research has indicated it's associated with more bothersome hot flashes in menopausal women. If trips to the bathroom are disrupting your sleep, limit how much you drink before bed.

6   **LIMIT DAYTIME NAPS.** Naps may help you feel more rested, but long naps can interfere with nighttime sleep. If you nap, keep the length to between 10 and 30 minutes, and don't take it late in the day.

7   **EXERCISE.** If you're tired, exercise may be the last thing you feel like doing. But physical activity can help you sleep better and more deeply and is a proven way to reduce fatigue. Given the benefits exercise has in reducing disease and perhaps managing your symptoms, it's a win-win! But ensure you time your physical activity earlier in the day so that it doesn't leave you too energized to fall asleep.

>> FOCUS ON PREVENTION

The time leading up to menopause is a prime opportunity to get a handle on your overall health. Work with your health care provider to ensure you're up to date with necessary screenings and implementing any recommended lifestyle changes that will allow you to sail into your postmenopausal years in optimal condition.

The essentials

1 **HEALTH CONSIDERATIONS AT MENOPAUSE.** The menopausal years are associated with a number of health changes. Some health conditions are directly affected by the hormonal changes at menopause, some are a result of aging itself, and others may be due to a combination of both. It's important to understand what conditions to be aware of as you age. Three in particular to be aware of are osteoporosis, cardiovascular disease and breast cancer.

What you can do

1 **STAY UP TO DATE WITH SCREENINGS.** As you approach menopause, ensure you are current with any necessary tests. The table at right lists recommended screening frequencies for healthy adults. Your own needs will depend on your health conditions, risk factors, genetics, family history and lifestyle. Work with your health care provider to determine your individualized screening schedule.

2 **BE AWARE OF OTHER CONDITIONS.** Talk with your health care provider and learn the signs and symptoms of other conditions such as heart attacks, stroke, ovarian cancer and uterine (endometrial) cancer.

3 **STAY INFORMED.** See Part Four of the book for more information on taking care of your health in menopause and beyond.

Health concern	Recommended screening frequency in healthy women
Blood pressure	Get tested at least every two years if your blood pressure is normal and more frequently if it's higher.
Breast cancer	Although there's disagreement about when to start breast cancer screening and how often to repeat it, Mayo Clinic recommends annual mammograms starting at age 40.
Cervical cancer	Women ages 30 to 65 should have a Pap test along with high-risk human papillomavirus (HPV) testing together every five years. A Pap test alone every three years is also adequate.
Cholesterol	Have your levels tested every five years.
Colon cancer and polyps	Starting at age 50, women at average risk of colon cancer and polyps should be screened every three to 10 years depending on the testing option they choose.
Diabetes	Women age 45 and older or any woman with high blood pressure, a body mass index (BMI) above 25 or additional risk factors for diabetes should have her fasting blood glucose level checked every three years.
Eye health	Get an eye exam every one to three years if you have vision problems or are at risk of glaucoma.
Oral health	See your dentist once or twice a year for a cleaning and exam.
Osteoporosis	Generally, only women over 65 should get a bone density test, but talk to your health care provider to find out if you are at increased risk and should be screened earlier.
Sexually transmitted infections (STIs)	If you're sexually active, talk to your health care provider to see if you should be tested for STIs.
Skin conditions	The American Cancer Society recommends monthly self-exams to monitor for changes to your skin, such as unusual blemishes or moles.
Vaccines	Vaccines aren't screenings, but they're an important preventive measure. Get an annual flu shot and make sure you are up to date with your tetanus-diphtheria booster, which is needed every 10 years.

❯❯ DE-STRESS

Midlife can be a busy and complex time. Your work, relationship and family commitments are likely rewarding as well as demanding, and the uncertainties and symptoms of menopause can add another layer of stress. But don't lose hope. There are many tools available to help you manage your stress and gain a positive outlook on life.

The essentials

1 **ARE YOU STRESSED?** Take a step back and assess your stress levels. Are you feeling overwhelmed and fatigued? Your muscles may be tight or your jaw may be sore from grinding your teeth or being clenched at night. Do you feel anxious or moody, or do you have head-aches and trouble sleeping? These are just some of the red flags that you might be under stress.

2 **STRESS IMPACTS YOUR HEALTH AND WELL-BEING.** Stress can make it more challenging to face the changes and symptoms of menopause. Stress is a significant contributor to sleep problems, and increased anxiety can worsen your hot flashes. The hormones your body releases when you experience stress can increase your blood pressure, heart rate and blood sugar level. Chronic stress can contribute to heart disease, obesity, depression and other health problems.

What you can do

1 **TAKE TIME FOR YOURSELF.** Good self-care is an important way to cope with life's stresses. Set aside time each day to check in with yourself. Organize your thoughts and to-do list so that you feel ready to tackle your commitments. Take a bath or enjoy a massage to relieve your tense muscles. Find a fulfilling creative outlet such as art or music. Reconnect with hobbies you enjoy, or try something new. Getting proper sleep, adequate exercise and a healthy diet can also help you keep stress in check.

2 **TRY RELAXATION TECHNIQUES.** Relaxation is invaluable for maintaining your health and repairing the toll that stress takes on your mind and body. Many relaxation techniques and practices — such as meditation, tai chi, deep breathing, yoga, visualization, progressive muscle relaxation and mindfulness — help you to slow down, refocus your attention and increase your sense of well-being. It doesn't matter which relaxation technique you choose. What matters is that you select a technique that works for you and that you practice it regularly. See Chapter 11 for further discussion of mind and body therapies.

3 **REACH OUT.** Talk to friends or a therapist, or join a support group where you can share your feelings with others who can relate to your experience. And talk to your health care provider about how you are feeling. Fluctuating hormone levels may cause some women to experience depression around menopause. You don't have to weather the storm alone — there are a variety of treatment options available to help manage stress and mood problems.

You've got this

Menopause is inevitable, but it doesn't have to be intolerable. Far from it! By following the five steps in this chapter, you'll be well on your way to feeling in control and empowered as you move forward through this life passage.

Menopause basics

CHAPTER ONE

What is menopause?

It may start with changes to your period. Perhaps they're not as regular as they used to be. They're heavier than usual, or lighter. Maybe you miss one completely. At first, you worry you're pregnant. (Wouldn't that be a shock!) But then, you get your period … two weeks later than usual.

Other changes start, too — subtle enough that you don't notice them at first. You're waking up at night, even though you've never had trouble sleeping before. You feel moodier, and occasionally find yourself snapping at your family or becoming annoyed with a co-worker. Your breasts are sometimes tender, you feel like you're having trouble focusing … and was that a hot flash?

You do the math and realize that, yes, you're about the age your mom was when she starting going through menopause. ("Is that possible?" you wonder. "I feel so much younger!") You talk to your sisters or girl-friends about their experiences. You look up the symptoms of menopause on the Internet. You go three months without a period. You think that this may be it …

… and get your period the next day.

A normal part of life

Menopause — which marks the end of your menstrual cycles — is a time of great change. It's also a healthy, natural and normal part of life.

By its simplest definition, menopause occurs when your ovaries stop making estrogen and progesterone — female hormones necessary to maintain your menstrual cycles and fertility. In most women, menopause occurs naturally, at about age 51. In some women, menopause may be the result of a medical procedure, such as chemotherapy, pelvic radiation therapy or the surgical removal of the ovaries.

Most women will notice changes in their bodies in the years before menopause (perimenopause) and after menopause (postmenopause). These changes, like menopause itself, vary among women. While some women experience many symptoms of menopause (including hot flashes and night sweats), other women experience few, if any, disruptions.

Each woman's menopause experience is unique. And while some of the changes you encounter may feel surprising or uncomfortable initially, take heart from the fact that what you're going through is a natural part of life — one that you, like millions of women before you, will be able to handle.

Don't worry. You've got this.

Hormonal changes during your lifetime

Throughout your life, hormones — chemical substances that influence other cells in your body — play a vital role in your health and development.

When you were young, low levels of the female hormone estrogen influenced the growth of your bones and muscles (not to mention your brain, heart and blood vessels). As you neared puberty, estrogen production increased and determined the start of your first period.

During your reproductive years, hormone levels fluctuate on a monthly basis. In fact, it's this constant rise and fall that controls your menstrual cycle. At the beginning of each month's cycle, for instance, estrogen and progesterone levels are low, and start to rise, thickening the lining of your uterus in preparation for an egg (oocyte). About 14 days later, hormone levels rise again as you ovulate — which is when the egg leaves your ovary and travels down the fallopian tube to your uterus. If you don't become pregnant at this point (because the egg is not fertilized by a sperm), hormone levels start to fall, and your uterine lining is shed as you have your period. This happens time and again, month after month, throughout your reproductive years.

As you age, however, and nears the end of your reproductive years — typically around your mid-40s — the consistent rise and fall of hormones

Hormone primer

Your hormones change throughout your life, playing important roles in reproductive health. Here's a look at the key ones.

▶ *Estrogen.* This female hormone, released by the ovaries, helps regulate the menstrual cycle during the reproductive years. Estrogen levels rise and fall during your menstrual cycle, and significantly decrease by menopause. Prior to menopause, estradiol is the primary estrogen in your body. After menopause, estrone becomes the dominant form.

▶ *Progesterone.* This female hormone, also released by the ovaries, stimulates the uterus to prepare for pregnancy and helps maintain a pregnancy. Progesterone levels drop after menopause.

▶ *Follicle-stimulating hormone (FSH).* This hormone, secreted by the pituitary gland, stimulates the ovaries to produce eggs. (In men, FSH stimulates the production of sperm.) FSH levels go up and down during your menstrual cycle and rise at menopause.

▶ *Luteinizing hormone (LH).* This hormone, also secreted by the pituitary gland, triggers ovulation. Levels of LH also rise at menopause.

▶ *Testosterone.* This male hormone, which belongs to a class of hormones called androgens, is also released in small amounts in women, through the ovaries and adrenal glands. Testosterone plays a role in your libido, and helps maintain muscle mass and energy. Testosterone levels go down gradually with age, and do not decline specifically because of menopause.

starts to change. Your ovaries, which produce estrogen and progesterone, get smaller, and their rate of hormone production becomes irregular and less predictable.

These hormonal changes — which mark the beginning of perimenopause — can cause irregular menstrual cycles and other symptoms, such as hot flashes and vaginal dryness. These fluctuations and changes may last several years before you experience your last menstrual cycle.

Eventually, the production of reproductive hormones slows to such a degree — and the number of eggs stored in the ovaries diminishes

Fluctuating hormone levels

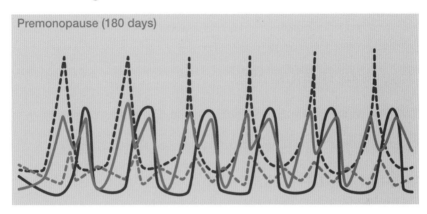

Premonopause (180 days)

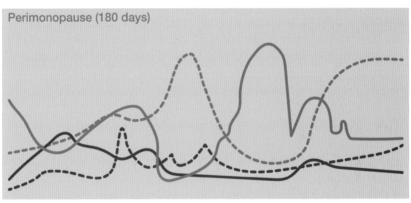

Perimonopause (180 days)

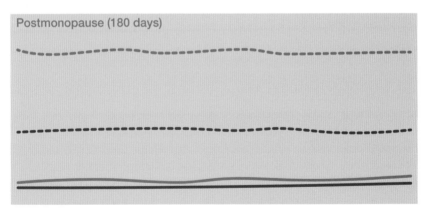

Postmonopause (180 days)

———— Estrogen   - - - - - - - Follicle-stimulating hormone (FSH)
———— Progesterone   - - - - - - - Luteinizing hormone (LH)

to such a degree — that your periods stop altogether. When this happens, and you have not had a period for at least 12 months, you have reached menopause.

Stages of menopause

Some life changes happen overnight. Others, like raising children, building a home or working your way up the corporate ladder, occur in stages, gradually over time. Menopause is in this group. In fact, the menopause transition typically has three parts: perimenopause, menopause and postmenopause.

PERIMENOPAUSE Many of the signs and symptoms that most women associate with menopause — from hot flashes to irregular periods — actually start in perimenopause.

Perimenopause, which translates to "around menopause," is the time leading up to menopause, or your last period. Women typically start perimenopause in their mid-40s (47 is average), though a wide range of ages — from the early 40s to early 50s — is normal.

Perimenopause is prompted by fluctuations in your estrogen and progesterone levels. The first sign of these fluctuations is often changes in your menstrual cycle. Initially, you may notice a longer time between periods, or notice that you are bleeding for more or fewer days than usual. Your menstrual blood may have more clots, or change color slightly. Hot flashes and night sweats also are common. Later in perimenopause, periods may

What is premature menopause?

Premature menopause is when menopause (whether it occurs naturally or is caused by medical interventions) occurs before the age of 40. Just as in menopause at the natural age, women who go through premature menopause quit having their periods and are unable to get pregnant. It's estimated that 1 percent of women experience premature menopause.

If you have stopped having your period before age 40 and don't know why, see your health care provider for further evaluation. Women who go through menopause prematurely are likely to benefit from hormone therapy to counteract some of the potential long-term negative health effects. Premature menopause is covered in detail in Chapter 2.

Menopause timeline

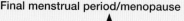

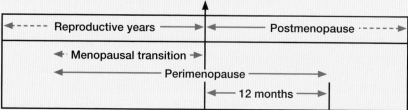

Adapted from World Health Organization. Research on the Menopause in the 1990's: Report of WHO scientific group. WHO Technical Series 866; 1996.

continue to change — such as appearing even further apart or closer together again for a time — and other symptoms may be added to the mix.

Perimenopause feels different for every woman who experiences it. A few lucky women will breeze through perimenopause and menopause without any bothersome symptoms. Some will experience the signs and symptoms for just a year or two, while others will be in perimenopause for nearly 10 years before reaching menopause. As a general rule, women will remain in the perimenopause stage for four to eight years.

Because signs and symptoms aren't always clear — and they may change from week to week and month to month — it can be hard to know exactly when you start perimenopause. If you're experiencing menstrual changes and other perimenopausal signs and symptoms, it's a good idea to talk to your health care provider. He or she can make sure there isn't another reason for these changes.

MENOPAUSE Menopause, interestingly, is a milestone you don't know you've reached until an entire year has gone by. That's because menopause — which is when your periods have permanently come to an end — is only considered official when you haven't had a period for 12 full months.

Why wait a year to make the call? Because some women, after going several months without a period, will think they've gone through menopause, only to be surprised by another period. However, once you've gone a full year without a period, you can feel confident that you've made the transition. On average, this happens at about 51 years of age — though there is a wide range of "normal," from the mid-40s to the later 50s.

POSTMENOPAUSE Postmenopause starts after your last period and continues for the rest of your life. For many women, this means at least one-third of their lives will be spent in postmenopause. (So it's fortunate that it's a fairly pleasant state in which to reside!)

Most women will tell you that the best part of reaching menopause is not having to worry about getting periods any longer. But there are other benefits, too. For instance, you also don't have to worry about getting pregnant. And many of the uncomfortable or bothersome symptoms you might have experienced in perimenopause — such as breast pain or mood swings — subside, as well. Your hormones will settle into steady, low levels instead of fluctuating like they did during your reproductive life.

Some of the symptoms of perimenopause — such as vaginal dryness or hot flashes — may continue into postmenopause. In fact, some women report experiencing hot flashes into their 70s. Fortunately, treatments and lifestyle measures are available to manage these conditions and help you stay comfortable and active.

Changes to the menstrual cycle

For many women, one of the first signs of perimenopause is a change in their menstrual cycles. This is primarily due to natural changes in ovulation (including changes in the frequency of ovulation) and hormone levels, including estradiol, the primary estrogen produced by the ovaries. No matter how regular or routine (or irregular and not-at-all routine) your periods have been historically, these changes can disrupt your menstrual cycle.

For some, the changes are subtle. For others, the changes are obvious — and disconcerting. Your period may come more often or less often. It may last more days or fewer days. It may be lighter, resulting only in spotting, or it may be heavier, bleeding through pads or even your clothing.

One of the most frustrating facts for many women is that all of the above may be true. One month, your period may arrive a week late and be lighter than usual. Then, just when you're about to celebrate this new development, your next period comes a week early and is so heavy that you wonder if you should buy stock in tampons!

For some women, these changes are no more than a minor annoyance. For others, heavy or prolonged bleeding can affect social lives, sexual relationships or stress levels. Less frequently, unusually heavy menstrual cycles may cause fatigue, headaches or anemia.

Changes in fertility

Your fertility, which is your ability to conceive a child, is at its peak in your 20s and declines with age. This decline typically starts after age 35 and continues through menopause.

Once you start perimenopause, it's more difficult, but still possible, to get pregnant. In fact, even if you haven't had a period in several months, you may still be able to get pregnant. It's only when you're postmenopausal that you can no longer conceive naturally.

For some women, reaching this stage of life can be an adjustment, and feel like a loss. Even if they had not planned to have more children, they may mourn the loss of their fertility. For others, the loss of fertility is a time of relief — a time to relax and enjoy unprotected sex for the first time in years.

Just be careful not to discard your contraception too soon. Make no mistake: Women can get (and have gotten) pregnant in the years and months leading to menopause. In fact, the changing menstrual cycles common during perimenopause can cause unpredictable ovulation — making it difficult to know when you are most likely to get pregnant, and putting you at risk of an accidental pregnancy.

Of course, this unpredictability can also make it frustrating for women who are trying to get pregnant as they enter perimenopause. If you are in this group, and are experiencing age-related infertility issues, there is hope. Medical interventions — such as in vitro fertilization (IVF) — can increase your likelihood of getting pregnant. If these interventions aren't possible or recommended for you, options such as using donor oocytes, a gestational carrier or adoption can help you build your family.

It may be reassuring to know that you're not alone — and that an end is in sight. Nearly all women (about 90 percent) who go through natural menopause will experience changes to their menstrual cycles. And, encouragingly, these changes will most likely be over in an average of four to eight years.

WHEN ARE MENSTRUAL CHANGES *NOT* NORMAL? Changes to your menstrual cycle are usually a normal part of perimenopause. In some cases, however, abnormal bleeding may require further evaluation to rule out a more serious condition. Talk to your health care provider if:

- Your periods become so heavy that you have to change tampons or pads every hour or two for two or more hours

- Your periods last longer than seven days, or several days longer than usual

- You are bleeding or spotting between periods

- Your periods are becoming closer together, regularly occurring less than 21 days apart

Your health care provider can help you determine whether these changes are a normal part of your perimenopause experience, or if they might indicate another condition.

What changes you might expect

Many changes happen to women as they enter midlife. Some of these changes are positive. For instance, many women in their 40s and 50s find themselves feeling more confident, self-assured and decisive than ever before. Some of these changes, on the other hand — such as those happening to your body and its systems — may be perceived as less positive.

Admit it: If you're nearing menopause, you've heard the stories. You've been told about hot flashes and weight gain, about mood swings and libido changes. You may worry about what's going to happen when you hit menopause — because if some of your friends are to be believed, it doesn't sound like something to celebrate.

The truth is, all women experience menopause differently. Physically, some women may notice only a few minor changes — some breast tenderness, perhaps, or the occasional hot flash — in the years before menopause. Others may feel as if their world has turned upside down as they manage night sweats, irregular periods and unpredictable moods.

You can read more about the changes you might experience during the menopause transition in the chapters that follow. Here's a preview:

- Hot flashes and night sweats
- Sleep problems
- Weight gain
- Mood changes

Personal story

Penny, 65

I guess you'd say that when it came to menopause, I was a late bloomer. In fact, there was a time when I wondered if it was ever going to happen for me!

In my late 40s and early 50s, I watched my friends go through perimenopause and, eventually, menopause — and there I was, still having periods. Every time I'd have my annual physical, my doctor would ask, "Are you still menstruating?" Grudgingly, I'd say yes, and he'd say, "Well, you know, the average age for menopause is 51, so somebody has to be on the high side to make that average!"

We had that same exchange, every appointment, for years.

When I finally did start perimenopause, at age 53, I really only had two symptoms: hot flashes and, oddly enough, regular periods — which, for me, were irregular. Ever since puberty, I'd had erratic menstrual cycles. I could go six, eight, even 10 weeks between periods. It never bothered me; in fact, I rather liked having infrequent periods. Then, at 53, I started having periods every month, like clockwork. It was like my body finally kicked in once I was ready to be done!

For years, I had hot flashes and those strangely regular periods. Then, as I neared my late 50s, my periods changed again. They started stretching out. I could go several weeks or even several months — and then only have a period for a couple of days.

I also started noticing other symptoms. Extra hairs began to crop up on my face. Extra weight settled in my belly. I had to cross my legs when I sneezed to keep from leaking urine (now that was fun). And my hot flashes became more persistent. There were times when I'd stick my head out the door in the middle of winter just to cool off!

I finally and officially went through menopause at age 58. (When I got what ended up being my last period, I remember thinking, "This is so wrong that I'm 58 and still doing this!")

The years since have been fairly anticlimactic. Sometimes I still feel kind of unbalanced. But for the most part, I enjoy being postmenopausal. It's nice not to worry about having a period. It may be one of the great perks of growing older!

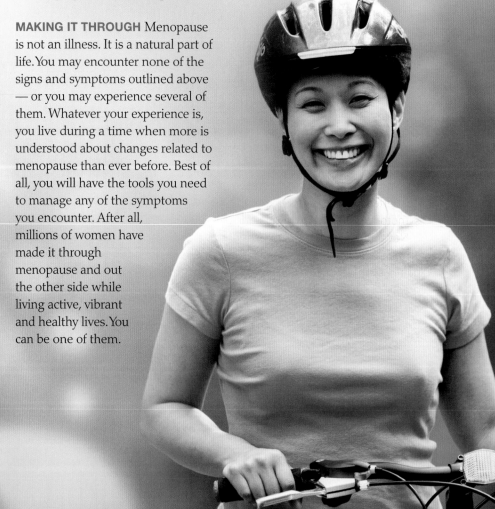

- Breast pain
- Vaginal problems
- Urinary problems
- Headaches
- Cognition and memory challenges
- Joint pain
- Changes to your hair, skin and eyes
- Hearing changes
- Dental concerns
- Bone changes
- Cardiovascular issues

Reading the list of menopause-related changes can feel discouraging. There's no denying that some of the changes to your body, and its organs and systems, can be challenging. But it's not hopeless.

MAKING IT THROUGH Menopause is not an illness. It is a natural part of life. You may encounter none of the signs and symptoms outlined above — or you may experience several of them. Whatever your experience is, you live during a time when more is understood about changes related to menopause than ever before. Best of all, you will have the tools you need to manage any of the symptoms you encounter. After all, millions of women have made it through menopause and out the other side while living active, vibrant and healthy lives. You can be one of them.

Personal story

Jennifer, 43

At 43, I still have my period. And, given my age, statistics say that I may have it for several years to come. But I'm definitely feeling the signs of changing hormones, and I have been for a while.

I was 40 when I first started getting symptoms, and at first I didn't realize what was happening. Menopause wasn't even on my radar. So when I started noticing more facial hair, mood swings and weight gain (after maintaining the same weight for two decades), I just figured that aging and a busy lifestyle were the culprits. Frankly, I'd never even heard of perimenopause.

In fact, when I started experiencing breast tenderness at 41, I thought, to my great surprise, that I was pregnant. After all, breast pain had been my first indicator of pregnancy with my sons 10 and 13 years earlier. I was so sure I was pregnant, in fact, that I bought a pregnancy test to confirm it. I was both relieved and confused when the test came back negative. (And, sure, maybe a little disappointed, too.)

Within a year, my periods became irregular. While they still arrived with the same frequency (about every four weeks), their makeup was unpredictable. One month I'd have a light period that lasted only a few days. The next month, my period would last a full week and be so heavy that changing tampons and pads felt like a full-time job.

I told my health care provider about my symptoms. I worried that something might be wrong with me. But after an evaluation, she said that I'd started perimenopause. I was surprised — but also relieved that my symptoms weren't a sign of something more serious.

Now, at 43, irregular periods and my other perimenopausal symptoms (like that cyclical breast tenderness) have become my norm. And while I can't say I necessarily enjoy the process, it really doesn't affect my life too greatly. It's just another part of my day, like attending meetings or driving my kids to activities. That said, I am looking forward to completing this cycle and going through menopause. Now that I'm on my way, I'm ready for the next phase.

CHAPTER TWO

When menopause comes too early

Rebecca, a 30-year-old advertising executive, started experiencing hot flashes in her late 20s. Her periods became very infrequent, as well, which was frustrating since she and her husband were trying to start a family. After undergoing some tests, she was diagnosed with primary ovarian insufficiency. Ultimately, they were able to conceive their first child using in vitro fertilization with a donor egg.

Sara, a single 34-year-old nurse, recently underwent a hysterectomy along with the removal of her ovaries and fallopian tubes after years of painful endometriosis. She's glad to be cured of her endometriosis, but worries about what the surgery means for her future health.

Andrea, a 41-year-old, stay-at-home mother of three, was diagnosed with breast cancer two years ago. After a mastectomy and several rounds of chemotherapy, she's in remission and back to living an active life with her busy family.

On the surface, these women don't appear to have much in common. But there's a common thread: They've each gone through premature menopause.

For most women, menopause occurs naturally at around age 51 — and it's rarely a surprise. By their late 40s or early 50s, most women have noticed the symptoms of perimenopause, and are watching for the signs of their final period. Some even welcome it.

Other women, however, follow a different path — a path they didn't plan for or anticipate. They stop having their periods in their 20s, 30s or early 40s. Women who go into menopause before age 40 are said to have premature menopause, a condition that affects approximately 1 percent of women. (Women who go through menopause between the ages of 40 and 45 are said to have early menopause. This condition affects approximately 5 percent of women.)

There are many reasons your ovaries might stop working early. Regardless of the reason, premature menopause is a manageable condition. This chapter will help you understand premature menopause, and walk you through the actions you can take to protect your health — and, if it's important to you, your dreams of building a family. You can live a fulfilling life with premature menopause. Let us show you how.

Premature menopause: Why it happens

Medical research has provided treatments and cures for more diseases and conditions than ever in modern history. Unfortunately, some of the treatments that can save your life can also damage your ovaries. If you go through menopause because of medical treatments, such as surgery, chemotherapy, or radiation, it's called induced premature menopause. If you experience menopause on your own before age 40 — as a result of health conditions, some genetic conditions or even unknown reasons — it may be known simply as premature menopause. But it may also be called primary ovarian insufficiency (POI).

SURGICAL MENOPAUSE Sometimes women, for various reasons, find they need to have their ovaries surgically removed during their childbearing years. Depending on the procedure, these women may experience different levels of menopausal symptoms.

If you have an operation to remove both ovaries (bilateral oophorectomy), for instance, you will stop getting your monthly period immediately, your hormones will drop quickly, and you will enter surgical menopause.

If you retain one ovary (unilateral oophorectomy), your body may continue to use that ovary to produce the hormones estrogen and progesterone. However, women who have a hysterectomy with unilateral oophorectomy before menopause may experience earlier menopause than do those who have a hysterectomy alone.

If, instead, you have surgery to remove your uterus (hysterectomy), but keep your ovaries, you will immediately stop getting your period and will be unable to become pregnant. However, you will not technically be in menopause because your ovaries will still continue to make hormones. This means you also aren't likely to experience any menopausal symptoms. In addition, women who undergo a hysterectomy may experience menopause up to four years earlier than the natural age.

If you do undergo premature menopause related to the removal of both ovaries, your menopausal symptoms may be stronger than they would be if you had reached menopause naturally. This is because in natural menopause, you experience a slow decline in estrogen and progesterone over time. But when your ovaries are surgically removed, you experience a sudden and immediate stop to your hormone production, including a portion of your testosterone production.

In surgical menopause, symptoms — such as hot flashes — may begin as soon as the day after surgery. Fortunately, there are effective options for managing these symptoms. Before surgery, talk to your health care provider about your treatment options.

CHEMOTHERAPY-INDUCED MENOPAUSE Chemotherapy is designed to attack and kill cancer cells. Unfortunately, this "take no prisoners" function may also damage your ovaries.

Not all chemotherapy drugs affect the reproductive system. Some may have no effect on your ovaries, others can cause a temporary stop of your periods or permanent premature menopause. Your risk of going into menopause depends on many factors, including your age, the kind of chemotherapy drugs you will be taking and the amount of chemotherapy used.

Typically any damage done is to the follicles — the fluid-filled sacs that hold your eggs. Women who've received chemotherapy may have decreased numbers of maturing follicles. While some women are not affected, others may experience menopause after a single dose.

Even if you do experience ovarian insufficiency due to chemotherapy, the condition may only be temporary. Some women — especially those under age 40 — find that their fertility returns months or even years after they complete treatment.

Considering oophorectomy

In some situations, such as treating ovarian cancer, removal of the ovaries (oophorectomy) may be a necessity. But in others — if you want to reduce your high risk of developing breast or ovarian cancer, for example — removing the ovaries as a preventive measure (prophylactic oophorectomy) may be a choice to consider.

Oophorectomy is not a decision to be made lightly. It carries significant risks. In particular, removal of both ovaries will cause immediate menopause. Common signs and symptoms of menopause, such as hot flashes and vaginal dryness, are likely to occur, and women who undergo oophorectomy often report their symptoms to be more severe than do women who go through menopause naturally. Oophorectomy may also increase your risk of conditions such as depression or anxiety, heart disease, osteoporosis, and premature death.

In addition, the procedure may take an emotional toll. If you have yet to have children or don't feel your family is complete, the loss of your fertility may be crushing. Some women also struggle with their sense of femininity.

That's not to say you should rule out the option. If your cancer risk is high, prophylactic oophorectomy reduces that risk significantly. If you're premenopausal with a BRCA mutation, prophylactic oophorectomy can reduce your breast cancer risk by up to 50 percent, and your ovarian cancer risk by 80 to 90 percent. The odds may make the potential complications well worth it.

The decision to have prophylactic oophorectomy is a challenging and difficult one. It comes down to a personal choice you alone can make. But advice from a genetic counselor, a breast health specialist or a gynecologic oncologist can help you make a more informed decision.

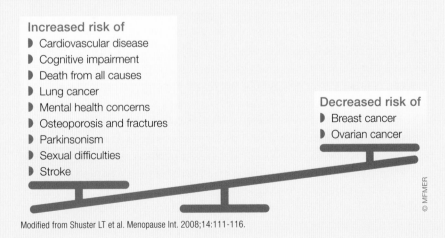

Increased risk of
▶ Cardiovascular disease
▶ Cognitive impairment
▶ Death from all causes
▶ Lung cancer
▶ Mental health concerns
▶ Osteoporosis and fractures
▶ Parkinsonism
▶ Sexual difficulties
▶ Stroke

Decreased risk of
▶ Breast cancer
▶ Ovarian cancer

© MFMER

Modified from Shuster LT et al. Menopause Int. 2008;14:111-116.

RADIATION-INDUCED MENOPAUSE Like chemotherapy, radiation therapy can be a highly effective method of fighting cancer. When this radiation is centered on your pelvic area, however, it can damage your ovaries. In fact, radiation therapy is typically more damaging to your ovaries than is chemotherapy. However, while chemotherapy is more likely to damage your ovaries' follicles, radiation is more toxic to the eggs.

Radiation's effect on your fertility depends on your age and the dose of radiation you'll be receiving. Radiation-induced ovarian insufficiency may sometimes be temporary, especially in younger women and in those who receive lower doses. These women may find that their periods return six to 18 months after treatment. Sometimes a procedure to move the ovaries outside of the field of radiation (oophoropexy) may be done.

OTHER CAUSES When something's not quite right in your body, it's natural to want answers. You may want to know what caused it, how it happened and how you can fix it. Unfortunately, when it comes to premature menopause, researchers and health care providers simply do not know the cause 75 to 90 percent of the time.

Some factors that may contribute to premature menopause are:

Genetic disorders Certain chromosomal problems — such as those involved in your reproductive hormones or ovarian development — can cause premature menopause. For instance, in a condition called Turner syndrome, women are born without all or part of one X chromosome, and, as a result, their ovaries may be underdeveloped. Turner syndrome is one of the most common causes of primary ovarian insufficiency.

Straight talk about primary ovarian insufficiency

Primary ovarian insufficiency (POI) describes what's happening in the ovaries. Whether their POI is due to genetic abnormalities or immune disorders, women with POI experience many of the realities of menopause — ceased menstrual periods, ovaries that no longer release eggs, a drop in estrogen levels — but not necessarily permanently. Their ovaries may still occasionally produce hormones and release eggs. Some women may even have an occasional return of their periods.

There also is evidence that women who carry the FMR1 gene — which is connected to a condition called fragile X syndrome — are at an increased risk of POI. These women may initially have regular menstrual cycles, even though their hormone levels more closely match those of aged ovaries. Many other genetic syndromes are associated with primary ovarian insufficiency. However, most are extremely rare.

Autoimmune diseases When you have an autoimmune condition, your body's immune system, which normally fights disease, actually fights itself. In some cases, such as in thyroid disease, lupus or rheumatoid arthritis, your immune system may attack your ovaries, preventing them from making hormones. This can ultimately lead to POI.

Metabolic disorders Certain metabolic disorders — such a galactosemia — may contribute to POI. People with galactosemia, for instance, are unable to break down galactose — a sugar found in lactose. Research shows that the defects in galactose metabolism may influence ovarian function.

Infectious causes Infections, such as mumps and HIV, may contribute to premature menopause by damaging ovarian tissue.

Family history If you have a family history of early or premature menopause, you are more likely to have early menopause yourself.

Addressing your physical health

When you go through premature menopause, your hormone levels drop significantly. Along with your reproductive life, estrogen loss affects:

Cardiovascular health Research suggests that early menopause may be associated with an increased risk of heart disease and stroke. This may be because of estrogen's effect on endothelial function, the health of the cells that line your blood vessels. For more on cardiovascular problems after menopause, see Chapter 14.

Bone health Estrogen plays a strong role in the strength of your bones. As a result, when you go through premature menopause, you have an increased risk of developing lower than normal bone mineral density (osteopenia) and bone loss that causes bones to become weak and brittle (osteoporosis). This is especially true for young women who go through premature menopause in their 20s, before their bone mass has reached its peak. You can read more on bone health after menopause in Chapter 13.

Cognition Some studies suggest that women who have their ovaries removed and who do not take hormone (estrogen) therapy have an increased risk of dementia and cognitive decline. The younger the age at the time of oophorectomy, the higher the risk of cognitive impairment. However, this risk hasn't been shown for all women who experience primary ovarian insufficiency. For more on cognitive issues and menopause, see Chapter 15.

Sexual health Low levels of estrogen can cause symptoms that may make sex uncomfortable. Women experiencing early menopause may also have lower levels of testosterone, which may negatively impact sexual functioning. For more on sexual health during and after menopause, see Chapter 7.

Quality of life Low levels of estrogen can be blamed for menopausal symptoms such as hot flashes, night sweats, vaginal dryness and mood changes. Read more about menopause symptoms in Chapters 3 through 8.

Help from hormones

All women who go through menopause — naturally or prematurely — may benefit from hormone therapy. Women who go through menopause at a normal age take hormone therapy with the goal of managing menopausal symptoms, such as hot flashes or mood swings. The reintroduction of

Could you be experiencing premature menopause?

Women who are entering premature menopause often don't realize it. That is because the signs aren't always clear.

A woman in the early stages of premature menopause may stop having periods altogether, or she may initially just skip one or two. She may have some of the symptoms of menopause — such as hot flashes or vaginal dryness — or she may not have any, yet. This is because, even if a woman has POI, her ovaries may still occasionally release estrogen and eggs.

So how do you know if the symptoms you're experiencing are the early signs of perimenopause, premature menopause or even a health problem?

Your best bet is to talk to your health care provider. If your periods change significantly (become noticeably longer or shorter, or vary markedly from your usual schedule), or stop altogether for three cycles before age 40, make an appointment for an evaluation.

It's important to be evaluated, since missing periods could be a sign of a another health concern. Plus, if you're experiencing premature or early menopause, you're at a higher risk of certain health conditions, such as osteoporosis and heart disease. Diagnosis can be a powerful tool — allowing you to take steps to make sure you stay as healthy as possible.

ovarian hormones into your body also may help prevent heart disease, protect your cognition and minimize vaginal dryness. And hormone therapy is vital for preventing bone loss in women who have premature menopause.

In women experiencing premature or early menopause, higher doses of estrogen may be required to treat symptoms and decrease risks associated with the absence of estrogen, compared with the doses required in women going through natural menopause. Most health care providers recommend that women with early or premature menopause take hormone therapy until at least the age of natural menopause — about 51 years of age.

Hormone therapy is not, however, a cure-all. While it does reduce or eliminate many of the negative health consequences of premature menopause, it does not eliminate them all. Mood changes and sexual function, in particular, are not entirely managed with hormone therapy during premature menopause. To learn more about hormone therapy, see Chapter 10.

WHAT ABOUT THE RISKS? Much has been written about the risks of hormone therapy. If you have premature menopause or POI, you may worry that the hazards of hormone therapy outweigh the benefits.

To help determine the cause of your symptoms or skipped periods, your health care provider may:

▶ Ask about any menopausal symptoms you've been having.

▶ Conduct a pregnancy test. This will make sure that any missed periods aren't due to pregnancy.

▶ Test your hormone levels. Blood tests can evaluate levels of a form of estrogen (estradiol), follicle-stimulating hormone (FSH) and luteinizing hormone (LH) to determine if they are in the menopausal ranges.

▶ Check for medical conditions that may be affecting your period. Blood tests may measure thyroid-stimulating hormone (TSH), fasting glucose, serum calcium or phosphorus levels — to name a few.

▶ Check your ovarian reserve. An anti-Müllerian hormone (AMH) level is a test that can estimate your ovarian reserve. A pelvic ultrasound can be used to check the quantity of eggs in your ovaries.

Don't let this concern you. The medical trials that revealed the risks of hormone therapy were conducted with older, postmenopausal women — not in women in premature or early menopause. Therefore, the results of these trials simply cannot be applied to these younger women. In fact, the risks of not taking hormone therapy can be devastating for this group.

The bottom line: If you have premature menopause, and you do not take estrogen, you have a much higher risk of dementia, parkinsonism, cardiovascular disease, osteoporosis, sexual dysfunction, depression, anxiety and death.

Coping with premature menopause

Going through menopause can be an emotional time at any age. You may mourn the loss of your fertility, worry about the symptoms, and feel anxious about the months or years ahead. It stands to reason that these feelings are even more intense if you go through early or premature menopause.

You may feel shocked at the diagnosis — certain that you're too young to go through menopause. You may feel confused, unsure what steps to take next. You may feel devastated over the loss of your fertility, especially if you had planned to have children in the future.

You may feel angry about the changes premature menopause makes in your daily life — the symptoms you might have to face, the hormones or other medication you may have to take. Experiencing hot flashes or vaginal dryness in your 20s or 30s may make you feel like you're growing old overnight — and aging beyond your friends. With all of these turbulent feelings, early menopause can be traumatic. It may lead to feelings of depression and anxiety.

What about testosterone?

Estrogen and progesterone aren't the only hormones that deplete during menopause. When you experience premature menopause, particularly if your ovaries are removed, you will also experience a decrease in ovarian androgens. Androgens are the male sex hormones, such as testosterone. For some women, a decrease in testosterone isn't a concern. For others, the loss of testosterone may contribute to problems with sexual dysfunction. This is because testosterone plays a role in sexual desire and arousal. As a result, some women may benefit from testosterone therapy, as well.

The good news is that you don't have to go through this alone. There are many resources available to help put your mind at ease and get the answers you deserve. Take care of your emotional and mental health with this advice:

GAIN PERSPECTIVE Going through menopause in your 20s or 30s might not have been part of your life plan. But that doesn't mean you can't still realize your dreams. Many women before you have gone through premature menopause and gone on to have healthy, productive lives — and even families of their own. You can, too.

GET ACCURATE INFORMATION Educate yourself about what's happening with your body. No question is a dumb question. Your health care provider is there to provide answers. If you go to the Internet for information, be sure to visit only reputable websites, such as those aligned with established medical institutions, such as *MayoClinic.org,* or those ending with *.gov.*

SEEK EMOTIONAL SUPPORT Ask your health care provider to recommend a counselor and support group. Support groups are made up of people who understand what you're going through, because they're going through it, too. They can offer the compassion and encouragement that others might not. And a counselor who specializes in premature menopause or fertility issues can help you gain a sense of control over your diagnosis.

GIVE YOURSELF SOME TIME Sometimes the greatest gift you can give yourself is time to come to terms with your diagnosis. It won't happen overnight. Allow yourself the space to come to accept it. You'll get there.

ALLOW — AND TALK ABOUT — YOUR FEELINGS OF GRIEF If you had planned to have children, it's natural that you will mourn your vision for your family. Have open communication as you manage your feelings. And allow yourself to envision a new dream — maybe one that includes in vitro fertilization with a donor egg or adoption.

Can you still have a family?

For many women, the dream of having a family has been lifelong. These dreams can feel threatened with the diagnosis of premature menopause.

If you had hoped to have children in the future, facing premature or early menopause — or even the possibility of it — may feel hopeless. But you don't have to give up hope. Many women who go through premature menopause go on to fulfill their dreams of motherhood.

OPTIONS THAT INVOLVE YOUR OWN OVARIES There are several options that utilize the ovarian function you currently have:

Fertility preservation If you're facing a medical condition or treatment that may compromise your fertility during your reproductive years and you hope to have children in the future, ask your health care provider to refer you to a fertility specialist. A fertility specialist can help you determine your best options for building a family. A couple of options he or she might recommend before treatment include:

Conceiving naturally with primary ovarian insufficiency: Is it possible?

You've heard the stories. Women who were told they would never conceive — maybe even women who'd struggled with infertility due to primary ovarian insufficiency for years — suddenly become pregnant. "It's a miracle," they say. "We didn't think it could happen for us."

Could it happen for you? The answer is a cautious maybe — but the odds are low. Research tells us that approximately 5 to 10 percent of women who go through premature menopause due to POI experience spontaneous remission and are able to become pregnant. So while there's hope, it's not a strong method of family planning. If your goal is to have children, your best bet is to consider the options in this section of the chapter.

If you'd like to explore your fertility options, ask your health care provider about the testing described on page 43. These tests can help assess whether pregnancy might still be an option.

Freezing your embryos (embryo cryopreservation) Embryo cryopreservation is when a specialist harvests your eggs, creates embryos with your partner's (or a donor's) sperm, and then freezes and stores them for future in vitro fertilization. Embryos can be stored for many years until you're ready to use them — giving you the chance to regain your health or wait for the time to be right. And when that time is right embryos can be thawed and implanted in your (or a surrogate's) uterus. Embryo cryopreservation can have high success rates, but it can be expensive.

Freezing your eggs (oocyte cryopreservation) Oocyte cryopreservation is when your healthy eggs are harvested, then frozen for future in vitro fertilization. In order to use these eggs in the future, a partner or a donor will have to provide sperm. This can be a successful approach to preserving your fertility — but there are a couple of caveats. The procedure can be expensive. And just as in trying to get pregnant naturally, there are no guarantees.

Oophoropexy Radiation can be an effective method of treating cancer. But, if you are undergoing radiation in your pelvic area, it can damage your ovaries and their ability to produce eggs. An oophoropexy can help minimize your risk of this damage. During an oophoropexy, your health care provider moves your ovaries out of the area to be radiated. This is done before any radiation treatment, through a minimally invasive procedure.

OTHER AVENUES If, like many women going through premature menopause, you were surprised by your diagnosis and didn't have the opportunity to take preservation measures, there are still ways you can have a family.

In vitro fertilization (IVF) with donor eggs Even if you aren't able to produce eggs of your own (and even if you no longer have your ovaries), you may still be able to become pregnant via in vitro fertilization with donor eggs. In this procedure, eggs are collected from a donor, then fertilized with your partner's or a donor's sperm, and implanted in your uterus.

IVF has high success rates in women who have gone through premature menopause due to primary ovarian insufficiency. In some cases, however, IVF isn't recommended. For instance, pregnancy can be dangerous for women with Turner syndrome.

Adoption Many women who are unable to conceive a biological child turn to adoption to complete their families. Adoption can be a rewarding and fulfilling way to realize your dream of motherhood. In fact, many women who pursued adoption say they now couldn't imagine building their families any other way.

Surrogacy You might consider using a surrogate — a woman who will carry a baby for you. In this situation, your surrogate will use her own eggs and will be artificially inseminated with sperm from your partner or a donor in order to become pregnant. You enter into an agreement that you are the legal parent or parents of this baby.

CHAPTER THREE

Body changes from head to toe

You are not imagining things. Your eyes are drier. Your skin is itchier. You're getting weird hairs on your face. And your waistline is thicker — despite the fact that you're eating less and hitting the gym more. These signs and symptoms are real, and they're part of the natural transition that your body goes through as your periods come to an end.

You were expecting hot flashes, right? Not joint pain and dry eyes? You're definitely not alone.

Many women don't even think about menopause when odd symptoms first appear. After all, many symptoms of the menopause transition start when your periods are still fairly regular, and many have no obvious connection to hormones. It's common to worry that something is wrong with your health, instead of recognizing changes as a normal part of the process.

As women live longer, researchers are still learning about all of the symptoms associated with menopause. But this is clear: The gradual loss of estrogen in your bloodstream is responsible for a wide range of changes throughout your body — not just in your reproductive system. This chapter details the physical changes that you may experience, from the more common to the more surprising. Once you understand all of the things that are happening to your body, you can decide how to manage them. Of course, you don't have to treat every symptom. In some cases, the only relief you need is the reassurance that what you're feeling and observing is perfectly normal.

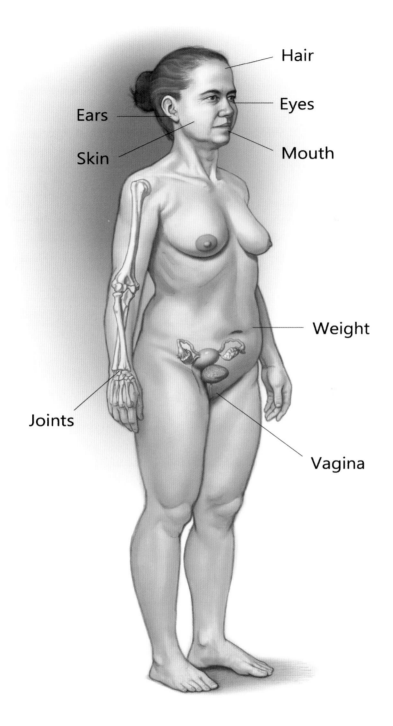

Hair

Eyes

Ears

Skin

Mouth

Weight

Joints

Vagina

Every woman's symptoms are different

There is no timeline or blueprint for the transition to menopause. Every woman walks through this transition in her own way. So it's impossible to predict exactly which symptoms you may experience or when they may creep up.

As you learned in Chapter 1, perimenopause begins years before your final menstrual period. Physical symptoms related to hormone changes often begin at this time — not the day your periods permanently stop. Women in all phases of perimenopause and menopause report a gamut of body changes. Some women are very bothered by physical symptoms that emerge. Others barely seem to notice anything different.

Whether you fit into the former group or the latter group — or somewhere in between — it's important to be aware of and informed about what's happening.

What's causing these changes?

The short answer is hormones.

As you approach your late 30s, your ovaries start making less estrogen and progesterone — the hormones that regulate menstruation — and your fertility declines. In the years before menopause, your hormone levels may rise and fall unevenly, dramatically and unpredictably. This causes your menstrual periods to become longer or shorter, heavier or lighter, and more or less frequent, until eventually you have no more periods.

However, these fluctuations don't just impact how many tampons you need to buy and whether you can get pregnant. Changes in your hormone production can set off a cascade of physical changes throughout your body.

Estrogen is a powerhouse. It is released into your bloodstream and travels to cells in many parts of your body — including your reproductive organs, brain, heart, blood vessels and bones. It plays a role in helping to regulate many bodily functions. When estrogen dips, you may feel it from head to toe.

At the same time, you may experience symptoms that aren't directly related to a decline in estrogen. It's not fair to blame your hormones for everything. Some changes in your body are simply due to growing older.

Your options for treating menopausal symptoms may be different from your options for treating symptoms that have nothing to do with hormones. Your health care provider can help you separate out your symptoms and manage them appropriately.

Symptom specifics

The rest of this chapter describes in detail the various body changes associated with the menopause years. Be warned: This list isn't very pretty. Some of these symptoms are unpleasant. But they are a natural part of aging.

Remember that you're unlikely to experience every symptom on this list in severe fashion. Plus, you'll learn how to manage any symptoms that bother you in upcoming chapters. (Note: Hot flashes and nonphysical symptoms — such as mood changes and changes in your sexual life — are noticeably absent from this list. They're covered in Chapters 4-8.)

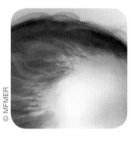

© MFMER

HAIR GONE WILD During the years surrounding menopause, it's common to find too much hair in some spots and too little in others. In fact, some studies show that approximately 70 percent of women who have been through menopause and didn't take hormone therapy during the transition develop more hair on their faces while losing hair on their heads and in the pubic region. It's common for these changes to occur during perimenopause, too.

Here are some of the hairy signs that you may notice:

Hair loss If you or your hair stylist has noticed that your hair is suddenly shedding or gradually thinning, that's perfectly normal. It may be time for a new hairstyle to help hide changes to your mane. Hair thinning during menopause can affect the top of your scalp, or you may develop a receding hairline along the top of your forehead.

That's because hormones influence hair growth. The exact mechanism isn't well-understood, but estrogen receptors are found on hair follicles. Estrogen seems to influence hair follicles in some way that relates to hair density. If your hair grew thick and fast during pregnancy — and maybe even changed texture — this connection will make sense to you. Unfortunately, you're on the flip side of hormone changes now, so you're seeing the opposite of those long, full locks you may have had during pregnancy.

Hair loss may also affect the eyebrows and pubic hair. In rare cases, women can develop patches of hair loss or near or total baldness.

Facial hair Hirsutism (HUR-soot-iz-um) is the medical term for unwanted, male-pattern hair growth in women. It results in hair on body parts where men typically grow hair, such as the face, chest and back. Many women experience facial hirsutism during the time of menopause — especially on the chin, upper lip and cheeks.

For some women, this manifests as fine hairs or peach fuzz, which can appear on larger areas of the face. Other women have lone, dark, quick-growing, rogue hairs that curl out of the chin or cheeks. In some cases, facial hair may grow to resemble a faint mustache.

The reason — again — may be related to a change in hormones. At puberty, your ovaries begin to produce a mix of female and male sex hormones. This is what causes hair to grow in your armpits and pubic area. Hirsutism can occur if the mix becomes unbalanced with a high proportion of male sex hormones (androgens). This commonly happens during menopause, as the ratio between estrogen and androgens shifts.

Hair changes can be mild or severe, inconvenient, or truly troublesome. Some hair changes may also be part of the natural process of growing older and not related to hormones. Your health care provider can help you understand your options for managing your particular signs and symptoms. If hair changes are affecting your body image and self-esteem, it's not vain or foolish to do something about them.

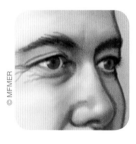

© MFMER

EYE CHANGES Sex hormone receptors have been found in many of the tissues of the eyes — including the colored part of your eye (iris), the clear elliptical structure behind the iris (lens), the protective dome of clear tissue at the front of your eye that helps your eye focus (cornea) and the transparent tissue that covers the white part of your eye (conjunctiva).

Researchers haven't determined the exact role of the estrogen and androgen receptors found in those areas. However, it seems that sex hormones are somehow involved in maintaining a state of equilibrium in your eyes. As a result, you may notice various changes to your eyes as hormones fluctuate throughout your life — during your menstrual cycle, during pregnancy and at the time of menopause.

Women report a host of eye complaints that occur with menopause. These include:

▶ Blurred vision
▶ Swollen and reddened eyes
▶ Tired eyes
▶ Trouble with contact lenses
▶ Vision changes

Think about your own eyesight. Do you find yourself holding books and newspapers at arm's length to read them? You might be experiencing presbyopia — the gradual loss of your eyes' ability to focus on nearby objects. It's a natural, often annoying part of aging. However, your ability to see may also be altered by changes or swelling in your corneas or other parts of your eyes as your hormones change. Many women find that they need reading glasses just before menopause.

Dry eyes One of the most common eye problems around the time of menopause is dry eye syndrome. Dry eyes occur when you can't produce enough tears to provide adequate moisture for your eyes. The medical term for this condition is keratoconjunctivitis sicca (ker-uh-toe-kun-junk-tih-VY-tis SIK-uh). Tear production tends to fall off as you get older. But women tend to report worse dry eyes and more severe effects on a daily basis than do men. This may be due in part to hormonal changes.

Dry eyes can be uncomfortable and distracting. If you have dry eyes, your eyes may sting or burn. Dry eyes can also cause scratchiness or an odd sensation that feels as if you have something stuck in your eye. A lack of tears in your eyes can also make you very sensitive to light (photophobia) so that it's difficult to drive or be outside without sunglasses. Environmental factors, such as wind and low humidity, can exacerbate the problem and make symptoms worse, so you may be more affected in certain seasons or as you travel to different climates. Some medications and conditions, such as rheumatoid arthritis and Sjögren's syndrome, also can worsen the problem.

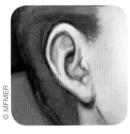
© MFMER

HEARING CHANGES Do you have a hard time hearing the conversation in a crowded room? Do you find yourself reaching for the remote to turn up the TV? Do you ask friends and family to repeat themselves, especially when talking on your cellphone or landline? You may be experiencing some changes in your hearing.

It's common to experience gradual hearing loss as you age. The medical term for this type of hearing loss is presbycusis. About one-third of people in the United States age 65 and older have some degree of hearing loss.

In addition, there is some evidence of a relationship among menopause, estrogen and hearing. Some researchers have found that estrogen may protect and preserve your hearing as you age. When you lose estrogen, you may lose some of your ability to hear right along with it. In addition, women who use hormone therapy to replace estrogen may have slightly better hearing than those who don't.

If you notice changes in your hearing, you may need to see your health care provider or an audiologist. Various tests may be used to quantify your hearing ability and look for evidence of hearing loss.

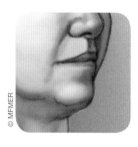

MOUTH AND DENTAL CHANGES Dryness is a recurring theme during menopause. You learned about dry eyes during menopause earlier in this chapter, and you've probably heard that vaginal dryness also can be a problem at this time. (You'll read more about this on pages 58-60.) But you might be surprised to learn that the drying effects of menopause can be prominent in your mouth as well.

The mucous membrane that lines the inside of your mouth (oral mucosa) contains estrogen receptors. So do the glands that produce your saliva (salivary glands). Estrogen seems to support the health of these structures in your mouth and plays an important role in keeping your saliva flowing. As a result, saliva production may trend down in step with estrogen production.

Is less spit in your mouth really a bad thing? Yes. Saliva washes away food particles, enhances your ability to taste and helps with digestion. Without a steady stream of saliva, you may notice the following oral conditions and problems:

Dry mouth Xerostomia (zeer-o-STOE-me-uh) refers to any condition in which your mouth is unusually dry. In addition to a parched, dehydrated feeling in your mouth or throat, you may notice bad breath, a changed sense of taste or lipstick sticking to your teeth. Dry mouth can be a minor nuisance or something that has a major impact on the health of your teeth, as well as your appetite and your enjoyment of food.

Burning mouth syndrome This is the medical term for ongoing or recurrent burning in your mouth without an obvious cause. The discomfort can affect your tongue, gums, lips, insides of your cheeks, roof of your mouth or widespread areas of your whole mouth. Symptoms may vary from mild discomfort to intense pain, as if you scalded your mouth. This condition is common in postmenopausal women.

Cavities As noted above, saliva helps wash away food particles. It also helps prevent tooth decay by neutralizing the acids produced by bacteria in your mouth. As estrogen and saliva drop, some women dread trips to the dentist's office because they count more cavities than ever before. Tooth decay can also cause tooth pain, tooth sensitivity, or pain while eating or drinking.

Gum infections Changes in your hormones may change the balance of healthy bacteria in your mouth. This can leave your gums susceptible to plaque and make it more difficult to fight off infection. Gum infections, such as gingivitis and periodontitis, are both common in post-menopausal women.

Gingivitis is a common, mild form of gum disease that causes irritation, redness and swelling (inflammation) of your gums. Because it's mild, you may not be aware that you have this condition. In contrast, periodontitis (per-e-o-don-TIE-tis) is a serious gum infection that damages the soft tissue and destroys the bone that supports your teeth. Periodontitis can lead to tooth loss, if left untreated.

If you're experiencing uncomfortable changes in your mouth or teeth, make an appointment with your dentist. The sooner you seek care, the better your chances of identifying cavities, gum disease and other dental conditions before they lead to more-serious problems.

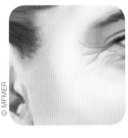

SKIN PROBLEMS A lot of magazine pages, television commercials and beauty products are dedicated to the idea of keeping your skin young. Anti-aging solutions for your skin come in all sorts of bottles, serums and syringes. So you're probably well aware that you may develop wrinkles, creases and sagging as you age. However, you may not be aware of all the changes to your skin that you may experience as your hormones change.

The truth is that hormones play a very important role in the health of your skin. The estrogen and androgens produced by your ovaries since puberty have nourished your skin for decades. Your androgen hormones help control oil production in your skin. At the same time, young skin is rich in estrogen receptors in the two outer layers — the dermis and epidermis — and it's clear that estrogen helps with a number of important jobs here. One of those jobs is metabolizing collagen — a fibrous type of protein that makes up your body's connective tissues and keeps your skin supple and pliable. As estrogen decreases, it greatly affects the amount of collagen in your skin, leaving skin thinner and wrinkled. Declining estrogen has other effects on the skin, too.

As your hormone levels change, you may notice a pronounced effect on your skin from your face to your ankles. If you think back, you've probably experienced changes in the appearance of your skin at other times in your life when your hormone levels made a major shift. Remember how your skin changed during puberty? Or during pregnancy? Or after you delivered a baby? Or when you tried a new birth control pill? Or even during your monthly menstrual cycle?

Here are some of the common skin changes that you might find during the menopause transition:

Acne It may seem completely unfair that you're growing older and reverting to your teenage skin all at once. Is it really possible to have wrinkles and pimples at the same time?

Unfortunately, the answer is yes. Acne occurs when hair follicles become plugged with oil and dead skin cells. When your body produces an excess amount of oil (sebum) and dead skin cells, the two can build up on hair follicles. They form a soft plug, creating an environment where bacteria can thrive. If the clogged pore becomes infected with bacteria, inflammation results. The plugged pore may cause the follicle wall to bulge and produce a whitehead. Or the plug may be open to the surface and may darken, causing a blackhead. If blockages and inflammation develop deep inside hair follicles, cystlike lumps can form beneath the surface of your skin.

It's very common for women who had acne in their teen years to experience an encore in midlife. This time around, lumps may be tender and appear deep beneath the surface of the skin.

The problem is androgen circulating throughout your body. As your estrogen levels drop, the ratio of androgen to estrogen in your body can shift. This can cause adult acne, particularly on the chin, jaw line and neck.

This problem can be distressing and frustrating. Be assured that effective treatments are available. They may just take a little time. You may need to work with a dermatologist to find a treatment that works for you.

Bruising In addition to keeping skin supple, collagen provides a protective layer between the surface of your skin and your blood vessels. As estrogen decreases and the amount of collagen in your skin changes, your skin may become thinner. As a result, slight injuries may be more likely to cause bruising as you age. You may notice more cuts, bruises and other marks on your skin. It may also take longer for these wounds to heal.

Dry skin Dry eyes, dry mouth, dry skin — you're seeing the pattern now, right? For some women, menopause feels like a drought.

Dry skin (xerosis) is a common condition of aging skin. For women, though, flaking and itching is very common around the time of menopause, as the production of skin-smoothing collagen drops. The changing ratios of hormones in your body also can affect the water content in your skin and oil production in your body, which can contribute to the problem. In addition, if the transition to menopause has you sweating a lot — such as soaking your sheets at night due to night sweats — your skin may be feeling the effects of all that loss of liquid and moisture.

You may notice parched, dry skin on your back, ankles, elbows, face or torso. It can cause significant itching and discomfort. It can also be aggravated by the climate or season. You may be the itchiest in winter or if you live in or visit dry climates.

Wrinkles Frown lines. Crows feet. Forehead lines. All sorts of wrinkles and creases can appear — or deepen — as estrogen declines. This is partly due to decreased collagen in the deep layers of your skin, causing skin to lose its elasticity and tone. In addition, decreased production of natural oils dries your skin and makes it appear more wrinkled. You may notice more-pronounced lines and crevices around your eyes and mouth and on your neck. Some wrinkles can become deep crevices or furrows.

You can't do much to reverse the hormone changes that contribute to wrinkles. But there are other factors that cause wrinkles that you can control. These include ultraviolet light, smoking and constant squinting. Avoid all of these things as much as you can. If the lines and creases on your face bother you, you'll find information about treatments in Chapter 16.

Other problems There are other skin changes and conditions associated with menopause. You may notice thickening of the skin on your palms and heels. Some women also develop rosacea (roe-ZAY-she-uh) at this time. This common skin condition causes persistent redness in the face and often produces small, red, pus-filled bumps. Signs and symptoms may flare up for a period of weeks to months and then diminish again before flaring up again. Rosacea can be mistaken for acne, an allergic reaction or other skin problems. Talk to your health care provider if you're concerned about other changes to your skin.

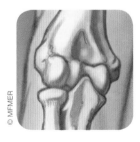
© MFMER

JOINT CONCERNS Joint pain is discomfort that arises from any joint — the point where two or more of your bones meet. Joint pain is sometimes called arthralgia or — particularly if inflammation or joint changes are involved — arthritis. The joint can feel stiff and achy. You also may feel some soreness each time you move the affected joint.

Joint pain and arthritis are common with age and are caused by wear-and-tear damage to your joint's cartilage — the hard, slick coating on the ends of your bones. This wear and tear can occur over many years, or it can be hastened by a joint injury or infection to the joint.

Women at midlife commonly report having joint pain, aches or swelling. Many women notice joint pain for the first time during perimenopause.

In fact, there seems to be some correlation between joint pain and menopause status. With menopause, women seem to be more affected by joint symptoms than are women who are still having regular periods. However, researchers are uncertain whether joint symptoms are related to a decline in estrogen or something else.

Some studies indicate that women with joint pain or stiffness may get some relief with hormone therapy. The relationship between joints and estrogen isn't fully understood, and more research is needed in this area.

However, if your knee feels stiff or you're having trouble getting your rings over your swollen finger joints, you can be reassured that these symptoms are common. At the same time, don't be too quick to shrug off new pain without investigating its cause, especially if pain is severe or impeding your activities. There are many reasons for pain in or around your joints. It's possible that your pain is actually radiating from the bone, ligament, tendon or the small sacs of fluid (bursae) that reduce friction between moving parts in your joint. Pain may also be traced to an injury or mechanical problem.

Your health care provider can help you sort out the cause of your pain and the best treatment. If the cause is an injury, hormone therapy won't be the right solution.

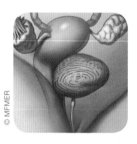

© MFMER

VULVAR AND VAGINAL CHANGES Your vagina is a muscular canal that extends from the neck of your uterus (cervix) to your vulva — the outside of the female genital area. The vulva is the area of skin that surrounds the urethra and vagina, including the clitoris and labia. The health of your entire female genital area — inside and outside — is an important part of your overall health.

Problems here can affect your desire for sex, your ability to reach orgasm, your relationship and your self-confidence. So it's important to recognize changes in this area due to menopause. For some women, these changes are all too obvious as shifting hormones can have a major impact on the vagina and vulva.

The following vaginal conditions are common during the transition to menopause:

Vaginal dryness Remember the dryness theme of menopause? In the early stages of perimenopause, you may begin to notice a slight decrease in the amount of vaginal lubrication you feel with sexual arousal and during sexual activity. This is often one of the first signs that estrogen is declining. As time goes on, you may notice a whopping dip in the amount of lubrication that you feel during sex. You may also notice vaginal dryness during daily activities, not just during sexual activities. Dryness may lead to discomfort and itchiness, too. All of these sensations are very common, due to declining estrogen and decreased blood flow to your vagina.

Genitourinary syndrome of menopause (GSM) This term is a medical name for the package of vulvar, vaginal and urinary tract changes related to the loss of estrogen. The vaginal walls may appear thin, smooth, pale and dry during a pelvic exam. This is a change from the way the vagina looks before menopause, when it's well-stocked with estrogen and the lining is thick and full of folds, allowing it to stretch during intercourse and child-birth. Vaginal dryness can be a symptom of GSM. Women with moderate to severe GSM may also feel vaginal burning, scratchiness or discomfort.

Most women experience some loss of fullness and thinning of the vagina during menopause. But, in some cases, it can be progressive and severe. As walls thin, the vagina becomes less flexible, more fragile and more susceptible to bleeding, spotting, tearing or pain during sexual activities or even during a pelvic exam. It can make sex very painful or even impossible. Changes to the vaginal tissues can also lead to infections. In addition, thinner vaginal tissues can be easily irritated, leading to redness, vaginal burning, vaginal discharge, painful urination, frequent urination or leaking urine.

All of these symptoms are the result of the decrease in estrogen production. As hormones shift, you may lose collagen under the skin near your vagina and urinary tract in the same way that you lose collagen elsewhere in your skin. As a result, the tissues of the vulva and the lining of the vagina can become thinner and less elastic or flexible.

Other factors can contribute to this problem, too. Smoking cigarettes or taking certain medications, such as antihistamines and antidepressants, can make things worse. So can a lack of sexual activity. In use it or lose it fashion, regular, *painless* sexual activity helps maintain vaginal health.

All of these vaginal conditions can understandably alter your desire for sex or enjoyment of sex. Estrogen also helps protect the health of your bladder and urethra — the tube that carries urine from the bladder. So changes in this area can cause bladder infections and urination problems. These problems are covered in detail in Chapters 7 and 8.

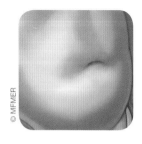
© MFMER

WEIGHT GAIN It's common for woman in the midst of menopause to swear that their eating habits and exercise routines haven't changed, but their waistline has. Even worse, many women say they're eating a healthier diet and working out harder and still gaining in pant sizes. What gives?

When it comes to your weight and menopause, you may feel as if someone suddenly changed the rules of your body and forgot to tell you. The eating habits and exercise routines that used to work for you may suddenly seem futile. Or you may feel as if you just can't cheat on healthy habits anymore — you can't skip a few days of exercise or binge on pasta and cake without seeing the effects on your bathroom scale.

These observations aren't off. The hormone changes that occur during the menopause transition can result in changes in your body composition, including an increase in the fat accumulation around the center of your abdomen. In practical terms, you may suddenly feel thicker or fuller around your middle. You may gain weight in your abdomen instead of your thighs and hips, and it may not budge easily.

Many women also gain overall weight during this time — about 5 pounds on average. However, it's unclear whether menopause is directly responsible for any extra pounds. Menopausal weight gain may be triggered by lifestyle changes that occur at this time, rather than hormonal changes. For example, sleep deprivation is often associated with weight gain. As a result, women who struggle to sleep well during menopause may pack on unwanted pounds, even though hormones aren't directly to blame.

Similarly, life events that occur at the time of menopause might change your diet or exercise habits and contribute to menopausal weight gain. For example, if you become an empty nester or undergo a divorce at this time, it may change how much you cook and how much you eat out. It may also have a significant effect on your weekly calendar and activity level. You may inadvertently bump up the amount of calories you're consuming or curtail the amount of calories you're burning without really realizing it.

Genetic factors also might play a role in menopause weight gain. If your parents or other close relatives carry extra weight around the abdomen, you're likely to do the same. Aging plays a role, too. As you age, muscle mass typically diminishes, while fat increases. When muscle mass decreases, it can decrease the rate at which your body uses calories and make it more challenging to maintain a healthy weight. If you continue to eat as you always have and don't increase your physical activity, you're likely to gain weight.

When you add up all of these factors, the math is clear: You will probably need to work harder to maintain your weight during menopause. Even if you're able to maintain your weight, you may carry it differently, and your clothes may not fit the same.

That's OK. There's no good reason to drive yourself mad trying to maintain a flat, bikini-ready stomach for the rest of your life. On the flip side, there's no reason to give up and resign yourself to an extra 10 or 20 pounds. Extra weight is associated with a number of health risks, including heart disease. So it's important to keep a focus on healthy lifestyle choices even more than your BMI as you age. You'll learn more about healthy lifestyle changes that can keep you feeling great as you age in Chapter 9.

Take action

For some women, understanding all of the changes that are happening to the body during menopause is a relief. It's a much-needed validation that what they're seeing and feeling is real and natural. For other women, this laundry list of menopausal symptoms is a bit daunting.

However you feel, the symptoms of menopause most likely will be your wake-up call to talk to your health care provider. Even though the symptoms discussed in this chapter are normal and natural, that doesn't mean you have to grin and bear them. Your health care provider can help you figure out a plan to handle any symptoms that you find uncomfortable or embarrassing. Unlike generations of women before you, you're living at a time when the transition to menopause is better researched and understood, and all sorts of options for managing symptoms are available. This includes lifestyle changes and traditional medications, as well as complementary and integrative therapies, such as meditation and more. Take advantage of the offerings that are available if you don't like some of the physical and emotional changes that you're seeing and feeling.

If you're among the lucky women who aren't bothered by any symptoms of menopause, that's great. This is a good time to check in with your health care provider and talk about a plan to keep it that way.

Symptom tracker

Date	Symptom	Level it bothers me (1-10 scale)	Potential triggers	Solutions I tried	New ideas to try

Questions for my health care provider

Before you see your health care provider, you may wish to write down any menopause-related symptoms that you've noticed. Tracking your symptoms for a few weeks can give you a clear record of how many symptoms you're experiencing, how often they happen and how much they bother you. You can keep a simple log on your mobile phone, in your planner or calendar, or on a scratch sheet of paper — anything that works for you. Whatever system you use, take your log with you when you visit your health care provider, and use it to talk through your symptoms and concerns. Then you can work together to develop an informed, thoughtful plan for helping you feel your best.

Finally, a word of caution: Take new symptoms seriously, and don't chalk everything up to off-kilter hormones. Although the transition to menopause can be responsible for a wide range of body changes and sensations, there are other serious conditions that can cause some of the same signs and symptoms — mouth pain, vision changes, bruising or joint pain, for example. It's important to pinpoint the cause of new signs and symptoms, particularly if they come on suddenly or are particularly severe.

Pay attention to your body, and keep in touch with your health care provider as things change. Don't overlook or downplay new symptoms by assuming that everything that happens to you can be pinned to menopause or aging. Menopause-related changes are just one part of your overall health. It's also important to consider your unique personal medical history, your family history, your health habits and other factors as you evaluate changes in your body. Menopause is just one piece of the puzzle.

PART TWO

Navigating the changes

CHAPTER FOUR

Hot flashes and night sweats

Most women experience hot flashes to some degree as estrogen production decreases significantly after menopause. In fact, about three-fourths of women in perimenopause or menopause in the United States report having hot flashes. This makes hot flashes the most common symptom of the transition to menopause. For some women, these temporary but recurring episodes of redness, warmth and heat are no big thing. For others, hot flashes are very intense, and more than a minor nuisance. These sudden waves of warmth can be annoying and embarrassing or even downright debilitating.

Plus, they can last for years. Accumulating research shows that health care providers have long underestimated the duration of hot flash symptoms. It had been widely believed that hot flashes would diminish and stop within a couple of years. But new studies indicate that many women experience hot flashes for an average of nearly five years after their final menstrual periods. When you add in the fact that hot flashes often begin several years before menstrual periods stop, that means many women are sweating it out for 10 years or more. (Yes, you read that right — a full decade.)

Keep this timeline in mind as you learn more about hot flashes in this chapter and consider the strategies or treatments you may need to keep yourself cool. If your hot flashes don't last that long, that's great. But it's better to proceed with the expectation that they could and seek solutions to find relief.

What is a hot flash?

If you haven't experienced your first flash of heat, you may be nervous or anxious in anticipation of this sensation. What is the hubbub all about?

You should know that hot flashes, hot flushes and night sweats are all the same thing. The only difference is that night sweats happen at night. The medical term for all of these symptoms is vasomotor symptoms.

A hot flash is simply a sudden feeling of warmth or heat that spreads over your body and is usually most intense around the face, neck and chest. During a hot flash, your skin gets flushed, red or blotchy, as if you're blushing. At the same time, you might start sweating — sometimes profusely sweating — on your upper body. Your heart may beat faster, too. Once the heat passes, you may develop chills or shivering.

A single hot flash typically lasts one to five minutes. They can repeat several times an hour, a few times a day, or just once or twice a month. How frequently hot flashes occur varies widely from woman to woman. But each individual woman usually has her own consistent pattern. In general, flashes become more frequent as your periods come to a halt. Hot flashes typically peak in the two years after your last period. Then, they decline with time.

A wide range of symptoms

Sometimes, flashes are mild, causing just a slight feeling of warmth. Others may leave you looking like you just stepped out of a Bikram yoga class. Night sweats come in the same range. You may sleep through some night sweats without noticing them. Others may be strong enough to jolt you from sleep in a sweat-soaked state that forces you to change your pj's.

Along with hot flashes and night sweats, women frequently experience other signs and symptoms. They may include:

▶ Irritability or anxiousness
▶ Difficulty concentrating or "brain fog"
▶ Fatigue, lack of energy or difficulty sleeping
▶ Feeling depressed or moody
▶ Impaired short-term memory

For working women, hot flashes can take a professional toll. New research shows that hot flashes account for a significant economic burden on working women and their employers. One study showed that women with untreated hot flash symptoms had a significantly higher frequency of doctor visits, absences from work and decreased productivity on the job when compared with women with no hot flash symptoms.

This isn't a revelation to any woman who has experienced hot flashes in the office, the boardroom or an important client meeting. Being red, sweaty, bad-tempered and unable to concentrate throughout the workday can have a major impact on your self-esteem, your social graces, and your professional drive and ambition. Even if you can shrug it off personally, it can undermine your authority if others misinterpret your symptoms as a sign of nervousness, insecurity or lack of preparation.

Hot flashes can also contribute to sexual problems and relationship strife. After all, hot, passionate, sweaty sex may have been a turn-on in your 20s. But, when hot flashes are the cause of all the heat and sweatiness, it may not lead to any burning desire. If you're struggling with night sweats, your bed may actually be a place of turmoil and distress, rather than a place of passion. You may also feel too tired and exhausted to think about sex.

All in all, hot flashes may be very disruptive to you, your daily activities, your family, your relationship with your partner, and your general quality of life. Simple sweatiness is only a small part of the problem.

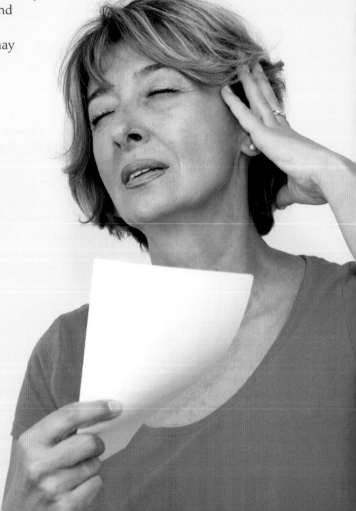

Risk factors for severe hot flashes

You may wonder how your particular symptoms compare with what other women are feeling. In general, doctors classify the severity of hot flashes and night sweats using these definitions:

▶ Mild. If you experience hot flashes and night sweats but they don't interfere with your usual activities, they're considered mild.

▶ Moderate. Moderate hot flashes interfere somewhat with usual activities.

▶ Severe. In this case, hot flashes are so bothersome that you have to interrupt or stop what you're doing to let them pass.

Researchers don't know exactly why some women land on the severe side of this scale and others don't.

Your risk of developing severe hot flashes depends partly on the following factors. Having one or more of these factors doesn't necessarily mean that you will develop severe hot flashes. But it's helpful to understand your risks.

YOUR STAGE OF MENOPAUSE The severity at which you experience hot flash symptoms is strongly associated with how long you've had them and where you are in the menopause process. If you begin having hot flashes while you're still having regular menstrual periods, the flashes may be mild at first. But symptoms can intensify over time, typically becoming the most extreme in the two years after your final menstrual period and then fading away.

YOUR EDUCATION OR INCOME LEVEL In general, women who didn't finish high school or have trouble paying basic bills tend to experience more-frequent hot flashes than do women with higher levels of education and income. More research is needed to understand this connection.

YOUR HABITS Many of your daily lifestyle choices and habits can impact your hot flash symptoms. Women who smoke are more likely to report severe hot flashes than are those who don't smoke. Similarly, women who are overweight or obese typically have more hot flashes than do women who maintain a normal weight. Physical activity can make a difference, too. If you don't get much physical activity for any reason, you may be more likely to have hot flashes during menopause.

YOUR RACE OR CULTURE Studies consistently show that black women are more likely to report having hot flashes and night sweats than are Hispanic or white women. Hot flashes are least common among women of Japanese and Chinese descent. This may be partly due to differences in biology or physiology, but the discrepancy may also be traced to differences in body weight, economic status, traditional cultural diets or other factors.

SURGICAL HISTORY Surgical removal of one or both ovaries (oophorectomy) is sometimes necessary to treat ovarian tumors or cysts, ovarian cancer, endometriosis, or other conditions. If both ovaries are removed before the natural age of menopause, it results in a sudden and immediate decline in the hormones that are produced by the ovaries. This surgically induced menopause can be an abrupt and much tougher transition than the gradual loss of hormones that takes place during natural menopause.

Severe or very frequent hot flashes may begin right after oophorectomy. In addition, women who enter menopause in this fashion may be more likely to experience other symptoms that can accompany hot flashes, including a depressed mood, problems with self-image and difficulty concentrating.

MEDICAL HISTORY Women who undergo cancer treatment — including radiation, chemotherapy or bone marrow transplant — may experience an abrupt decline in estrogen. This quick shift can result in severe hot flash symptoms, similar to surgical removal of the ovaries.

In addition, many cancer medications, including tamoxifen and aromatase inhibitors, can worsen hot flash symptoms. Tamoxifen may be used before or after menopause as an additional therapy to keep cancer from returning. For women at high risk of breast cancer, tamoxifen may also be prescribed as a preventive therapy to keep cancer at bay. In contrast, aromatase inhibitors are only used after menopause. This class of medications reduces the amount of estrogen in the body after menopause to help keep cancer from returning. All of these medications can be good for cancer, but bad for hot flashes.

Finally, women with a history of breast cancer may have more trouble with hot flashes because they may not be able to take hormone therapies that can help ease symptoms. However, other treatments may be helpful.

What causes hot flashes?

The exact cause of hot flashes isn't fully understood. But researchers believe that a part of the brain called the hypothalamus is involved.

The hypothalamus produces hormones that regulate a number of functions in your body, including your hunger and thirst. But one of the main jobs of the hypothalamus is to keep your core body temperature between an upper threshold (at which you'll sweat) and a lower threshold (at which you'll shiver).

When your hypothalamus is functioning properly, you're like Goldilocks — not too hot and not too cold, but just right. In scientific terms, the "just-right" zone is known as the thermoneutral zone.

As estrogen declines, this zone seems to narrow, and the hypothalamus seems to grow more sensitive to slight changes in your body temperature. As a result, your hypothalamus may overreact to any small rise in your core body temperature — such as when you sit in a sunny room or drink a hot coffee. The hypothalamus senses this extra warmth and mistakenly believes that you're too hot. It starts a chain of events to cool you down, which includes opening blood vessels near the surface of your skin to increase blood flow and release heat. Ironically, the hypothalamus's overeager attempt to dissipate heat results in sudden warmth, flushing and sweating.

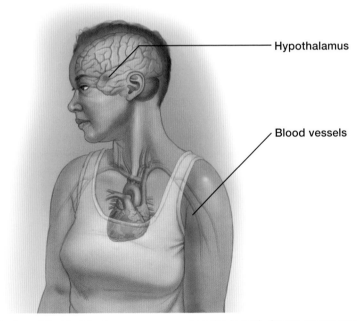

Hypothalamus

Blood vessels

It's believed that hot flashes may occur when the hypothalamus grows more sensitive to slight changes in your body temperature. This starts a chain of events to cool you down, which includes opening blood vessels near the surface of your skin to increase blood flow and release heat.

More research is needed to pinpoint the exact mechanism of hot flashes. Better understanding of the underlying process will help scientists create newer, better treatments for hot flashes.

Temperature triggers

Hot flashes may seem unpredictable and erratic. Even if you've been experiencing hot flashes for a while, their appearance may continually take you by unwelcome surprise. However, for many women, there are predictable triggers. Learning your triggers can help you find relief.

As you learned above, hot flashes may be partly due to your body's faulty reaction to a minor boost in your body temperature. So it's no surprise that many common triggers of hot flashes cause your body temperature to spike temporarily. In your younger years, these triggers wouldn't cause any concern. But, now, they cause your body to feel too warm and signal the sequence of events that leads to a hot flash. Here are some common culprits:

▶ **Spicy foods**. Blazing Buffalo wings. Fiery Thai noodles. Hot salsas. Sushi with wasabi. When your tongue is on fire from spicy foods such as these, it can spark a hot flash. Even if you like your food highly spiced, your body may sense a rise in temperature and feel the need to cool down.

▶ **Certain beverages.** Many researchers have looked at the connection between caffeine and hot flashes with mixed results. A recent Mayo Clinic study found that postmenopausal women who drank caffeinated beverages — such as coffee, tea or soda — experienced more bothersome hot flashes and night sweats than did postmenopausal women who didn't use caffeine. Alcoholic beverages also can be a problem. If you regularly consume wine, beer or cocktails and you're troubled by hot flashes, pay attention to see if this may be a trigger for you.

▶ **Smoking.** If you need another reason to quit smoking cigarettes, this is it. Both current smoking and a history of smoking have been linked to an increased risk of hot flashes. If you smoke, your hot flash risk may increase with the number of cigarettes or packs that you smoke. The exact relationship among smoking, nicotine and hot flashes isn't fully understood. It's possible that smoking has an effect on the way that your body metabolizes estrogen. Whatever the connection, it's clear that smoking worsens hot flashes.

▶ **A warm environment.** As estrogen declines and your body thermostat becomes more sensitive, you may find that you're only comfortable in a small temperature range. Any environment that's too warm can trigger a hot flash. The same is true of hot, constrictive clothing, warm bedding or other things in your environment that push you out of your comfort zone.

▶ **Stress.** It's tough to stay cool under fire — particularly during menopause. It's possible for a stressful situation — such as a contentious meeting or traffic jam — to trigger a hot flash. Women who experience ongoing stress may also be more likely to have more-frequent hot flashes.

FINDING YOURS Take some time to think about your triggers. If you're not sure, consider tracking your hot flashes for a few weeks. Make sure to log any possible triggers that might be related to your symptoms. Then, you can review your log and see if you can unearth any patterns.

You may find that your love of hot sauce plays a prominent role in your symptoms. Or that hot, stuffy meeting room in the corner of your office building is to blame. Or wool sweaters. Or too much wine. Or not enough stress-busting yoga. These insights are powerful.

How to get relief

If your hot flashes are mild, you may be able to manage them by revamping your environment and avoiding your triggers. If you experience moderate or severe hot flashes, keeping physically active and controlling your weight also can make a big difference. You'll also want to read up on medications and complementary therapies that can help. (See Chapters 10 and 11.)

Making over your surroundings and steering clear of triggers is a good place to start. Experiment with the following strategies and tips:

KEEP YOUR CORE BODY TEMPERATURE AS COOL AS POSSIBLE This seems like simple common sense, but it's hugely important in preventing hot flashes. Your goal is to keep your body temperature under your body's sweating threshold that triggers a hot flash. And, remember, this threshold may be much lower than it used to be. You may need to alter your habits and your wardrobe to avoid exceeding your limit.

Start by thinking about how you can remain in cooler, air-conditioned areas as much as possible. Open windows and use fans to keep cool air flowing. Lower room temperatures, if you can.

If you work in an office building, for example, intentionally schedule meetings in cooler, larger conference rooms or open areas. Don't pack into a cube or tight office space to discuss an issue. In addition, avoid back-to-back meetings on opposite sides of the building, causing you to rush from one area to the other. If you typically meet colleagues for lunch at an outdoor cafe or picnic area, look for shade or seek out a cooler indoor spot. Ask a trusted administrative assistant or colleague to help in any way possible. It may be embarrassing to discuss your hot flashes with colleagues, but it's better than the sweaty alternative.

Outside the office, plan your social gatherings at breezy restaurants or theaters that aren't hot and overcrowded. Or entertain guests in your own home, where you can control the temperature. When you know you'll be outdoors — such as watching your daughter's or grandson's soccer game — pack an umbrella to shade yourself from the sun. Whatever your daily routine, plan ahead and think of creative ways to keep cool.

In addition, get smart about your outfit choices. You may want to avoid a turtleneck or bulky dress. As much as possible, dress in layers so that you can remove a layer or two when you're hot and replace them when you're cooler. Try a jacket or cardigan over a sleeveless dress, silk shell or T-shirt that you don't mind showing off. Choose light, natural, breathable fabrics and open-weave materials that allow air to circulate.

Finally, carry a cool drink with you, when appropriate. If you feel a hot flash coming on, take a few sips or wrap your hands around the icy exterior to help cool you down.

KEEP COOL AT NIGHT If night sweats bother you, you'll need to find strategies to stay cool while you're sleeping — or lying in bed not sleeping, as the case may be. Start by surveying your bedroom. Is the temperature too high? Can you turn down the thermostat in the bedroom? Can you open windows or plug in a bedside fan for some breeze?

Next, examine your bed. Is it made up with flannel sheets and a huge down comforter? Or do you have multiple layers of breathable bedding that can be pulled up or down as needed? Wicking sheets could help, too.

Beyond your bed, make sure you have comfortable, light pajamas. And consider keeping a cold glass of water on your nightstand.

If you sleep with a partner, try to find cooling solutions that don't drive a wedge in between you. Hot flashes can be tough on your relationship. Complaining about your partner's body heat, throwing covers on and off all night long, or freezing your partner into the guest room won't help build any intimacy. Instead, look for solutions that keep you cool without icing out your partner. Try keeping a frozen cold pack under your pillow on your side of the bed. Turn your pillow often so that your head is always resting on a cool surface without affecting your partner. You may also find that cooling products — such as sprays, gels or special pillows — may be helpful.

WATCH WHAT YOU EAT AND DRINK Hot spicy foods are a common trigger for hot flashes. Keep this in mind if you're about to order zesty ribs, jambalaya, kung pao chicken, vindaloo curry or other fiery favorites. If you like bold flavors, look for dishes with fresh herbs, pungent cheeses, pickled vegetables or other ingredients that add taste and tang without adding heat and spice.

Mind your beverages, too. Hot drinks, caffeinated drinks and alcoholic drinks can all be a problem when you're trying to avoid hot flashes. Experiment with having your coffee at home before you shower, rather than saving it for the office. Swap caffeinated tea for herbal tea. Or try cold sparkling water or a refreshing fruit-and-vegetable smoothie instead of an afternoon soda.

It may take a little trial and error to find what works best for you. You may find that you can enjoy a steaming-hot latte without a hot flash, as long as it's decaf. Or you may find that coffee is OK as long as it's iced instead of heated. Find the limits that keep you comfortable.

REFRAIN FROM SMOKING Keep cigarettes out of your home and car. By not smoking, you may reduce hot flashes, as well as your risk of many serious health conditions, such as heart disease, stroke and cancer. If you need help quitting, talk to your health care provider about the best way to go smoke-free for good.

REDUCE YOUR STRESS Finding ways to reduce your load or increase the feeling of calm and balance in your life can help with hot flashes. Try meditation, yoga, massage or whatever stress-busting activities sound good to you. Even if these approaches don't quell your hot flashes, they may provide many other benefits, including better sleep.

If you're overwhelmed by stress or anxiety, seek support. Menopause can correspond with a lot of major life changes and transitions. Some of these changes are thrilling — such as watching your kids graduate from high school or college, planning your son's or daughter's wedding, welcoming your grandbabies, or landing a big promotion at work. Other common changes during this time are difficult — such as caring for aging parents or dealing with the financial stress of growing older and planning for retirement. In all cases, big life events — even the happiest ones — can cause stress. If you're struggling to manage it all, don't be afraid to lean on a good friend, family member or your health care provider. Getting your stress under control is important for your health. And you'll be able to better manage all of your responsibilities when you're feeling your best.

What to do when a hot flash is starting

Even if you make over your environment and do your best to avoid triggers, you may still experience hot flashes. When you feel a hot flash coming on, try paced breathing.

This type of breathing is slow, deep diaphragmatic breathing. With normal breathing, you take about 12 to 14 shallower breaths a minute. With paced breathing, you take only five to seven breaths a minute. And the paced breaths are intentionally slow, smooth and deep enough to move your diaphragm — the muscular wall located beneath your lungs. The goal of paced breathing is to reduce the stress chemicals that your brain processes and bring about a relaxation response within your body.

You can switch to paced breathing wherever you are when you feel a hot flash beginning — at home, at a friend's home, during a work meeting, in the car. Nobody even needs to know you're doing it. But it may take some practice to get the hang of the technique.

To practice diaphragmatic breathing, sit or stand comfortably with your hand on your belly and pay attention to your breathing. Imagine filling a cup with water when you inhale. As if filling a cup from the bottom up, fill your lower lungs and then your upper lungs by expanding your belly and moving your diaphragm. Pay attention to the movement of your belly under your hand as you inhale. During exhalation, reverse the process and empty the cup from the top down. Empty your upper lungs first and then the lower lungs.

Once you're comfortable with diaphragmatic breathing, focus on establishing a slow rhythm or pace. To start, you might try to make each inhalation and exhalation last for four or five seconds. You may need to count as you breathe in and out. (Breathe in, 2, 3, 4. And breathe out, 2, 3, 4. In, 2, 3, 4. Out, 2, 3, 4.) Over time, slow your breathing into a comfortable pace that equals out to five to seven breaths a minute.

If you need help learning this technique, you can teach yourself with an app, podcast or Web-based program. You can also seek the help of an expert to work with you in person.

A Mayo Clinic study shows that practicing paced breathing twice a day for 15 minutes seems to be most helpful, rather than just reverting to this technique in the throes of a heat wave. This breathing exercise is a nice, relaxing way to start and end your day. If you get in the habit of practicing paced breathing before you brush your teeth every morning and night, it will become part of your routine. You can also practice paced breathing as part of your cool-down after a workout, or you can take a paced-breathing break during your lunch hour. Find a time that works best for you.

Strike a balance

In the end, your goal isn't to stop living a full life — seeking out air conditioning at all costs while consuming only water and bland food. The point of understanding triggers for hot flashes is to seize control and feel your best.

You don't necessarily have to kick your morning cup of coffee. But if you're having bothersome hot flash symptoms and you're drinking caffeine, it might be worth considering cutting down a bit to see if it has an effect on your symptoms. The same is true of the other triggers. Identify your individual triggers and then use this powerful information to your advantage.

If you're unable to control your hot flashes by modifying your environment and avoiding triggers, talk to your health care provider about other options, including hormone therapies that can help. Remember that your symptoms could last for a decade. That's too long to rely on middle-of-the-night cold showers and a bag of frozen peas for relief.

CHAPTER FIVE

Moods and you

From the time you were an adolescent to today, hormones have been affecting your moods. This is because hormones — which are substances released into your blood by your ovaries and other glands — affect the chemicals in your brain that control mood.

During puberty, your hormones might've made you feel more emotional — sending you stomping to your room after a fight with your parents.

Before each menstrual period, your hormones might've played a role in increasing your irritability — causing you to snap at your children or become irrationally annoyed at co-workers.

During or after pregnancy, fluctuating hormones might've sent you on a roller coaster of emotions as you cried over the beauty of your new child while simultaneously panicking about the responsibilities ahead of you.

And, now, as you head into menopause, your changing hormones may, once again, be affecting your moods. However, hormones often aren't the only culprits. This chapter will explore the many causes of menopause-related mood changes, and how you can manage them successfully.

Mood changes during menopause

During your reproductive years, you may have noticed the connection between your mood and your menstrual cycles. Perhaps you felt slightly more emotional just before your period, or maybe you could go so far as to predict the start of your period based on mood alone. These mood-related menstrual symptoms — known as premenstrual syndrome (PMS) — are common.

As you head into menopause, you might've hoped that any mood swings associated with your menstrual cycle would be over. Unfortunately, this isn't always the case. Some women find that they continue to experience moodiness as they transition to menopause. In fact, research suggests that some anxiety symptoms, such as nervousness and worry, occur more frequently during perimenopause than at any time before it. These mood swings may be frequent or occasional. They may seem cyclical, like those during your reproductive years, or they may just leave you feeling generally more emotional or irritable.

The mood swings associated with menopause often aren't predictable. One day, you're laughing with your partner as you make plans for the future. The next day, you're crying over a greeting card commercial and snapping at your partner over, literally, spilled milk.

Part of the blame can certainly go to hormone fluctuations. As you transition through menopause, your estrogen levels become erratic — rising and falling (and then falling some more) as your body changes. These changing hormone levels may cause the irritability, tension, worry, anxiety and feelings of despair that are also associated with PMS.

However, mood changes may also be caused by changes that are happening in your life. For instance, many of the changes that happen around midlife — such as aging parents, growing children and planning for your own future — can be stressful and overwhelming. You may be sad over the loss of your fertility, worried about growing older and wonder what's next for you. It's no surprise that feelings like these can lead to stress, anxiety or a depressed mood.

Other factors that may affect your mood during menopause include:

▶ Severe menopausal symptoms. Sleep problems, hot flashes and menopause-related fatigue can affect your mood.

▶ Nervous or unsure feelings about menopause. You may worry about your changing body and what that means for you.

▶ Feelings about fertility. You may be sad about not being able to have more children — even if you considered your family complete.

▶ Poor health habits, including smoking, lack of exercise and a poor diet.

▶ Relationship troubles. Relationships with your partner, children or parents may be in transition during this time. Some women may go through the death of a loved one or a divorce.

▶ A lack of strong social connections. After years of raising children, you may find yourself alone or with a smaller network of friends.

▶ Changes in employment or income. A change in employment or the prospect of retirement can weigh heavily on your moods.

Whatever the reason, there are actions you can take to adapt to the changes in your life and overcome some mood swings. For instance, getting enough sleep, eating a healthy diet and keeping up with a regular exercise program can go a long way for your mental health. And adopting a positive attitude can make a big difference, too. Instead of looking at menopause for what you've lost, for instance, try to look at what you've gained. This time of life can be a great time to explore new opportunities, spend more time with your partner or friends, and really define what you want your life to look like.

Sometimes the mood changes associated with menopause are more severe — resulting in depression or overwhelming stress. In these cases, coping mechanisms such as adopting a healthy lifestyle and a positive attitude aren't enough. We'll explore these more-serious conditions below — along with ways to manage them.

Depression during menopause

Everybody feels sad from time to time. You get in a fight with your partner, a dear friend moves away, you miss out on that promotion at work. You feel terrible — maybe for a couple of hours, maybe for a couple of days — but are able to continue on with your life.

Depression is different. Depression is a serious mood disorder that interferes with your daily life. The feelings of sadness and hopelessness that accompany depression are so severe that you may not feel like eating, going to work or even getting out of bed. Depression can affect your relationships, your job and your physical health.

A combination of factors — genetic and chemical, environmental and psychological — appear to play a role in whether someone develops depression. Lifestyle changes, such as illnesses, work or family changes, or even severe menopause symptoms can lead to feelings of sadness and despair, too. Some women may have trouble coming to terms with losing their fertility, growing older and facing mounting menopausal symptoms. For some, it can be hard to bounce back.

Hormones, which affect the chemicals in your brain that control your mood, also may contribute to depression. It's not clear exactly what role these hormones play. However, research does suggest that menopause-aged women — and, specifically, women in the perimenopause stage — are at an increased risk of depression. This may be, in part, because of the amount of hormone changes occurring in your body as it begins the transition to menopause. (On the bright side, once you go through menopause and are considered postmenopausal, the risk of depression goes down.)

It's important to note that most women transition to menopause without experiencing depression — or any other major mental disorder. In fact, some women don't experience any mood changes whatsoever. You may be one of these women. However, you should be aware of your risks, and the signs and symptoms of depression, so you know what to look for in order to get help, if necessary.

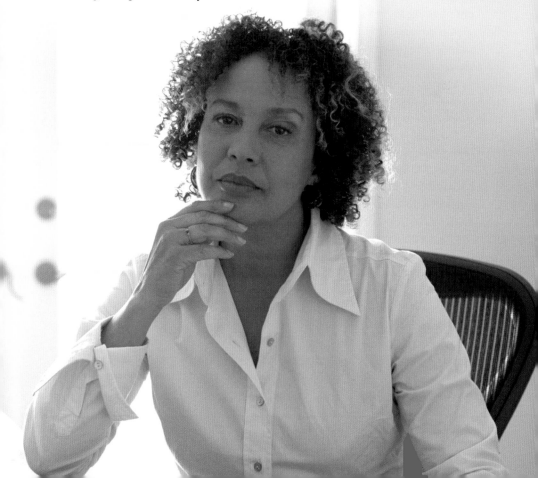

Women with a history of hormone-related mood changes are at a higher risk of developing depression during menopause. And women who have a mood disorder, such as depression, bipolar disorder or schizophrenia, are more likely to have issues at this time, as well. Other factors that can increase your risk of depression include high stress or having experienced stressful life events during childhood.

What depression looks and feels like varies from woman to woman, and can range from mild to severe. Common signs and symptoms may include:

▶ Sad, hopeless or negative feelings. In depression, these interfere with daily life and don't go away.

▶ Feeling anxious, irritable or restless. Or you may feel helpless or worthless.

▶ Losing interest in activities that you once enjoyed. This might include spending time with friends, pursuing hobbies or even sex.

▶ Fatigue. You may feel this way even after a good night's sleep or even after getting more sleep than usual.

▶ Changes in your eating habits. Either overeating or losing your appetite can be a symptom of depression.

▶ Physical problems. These may include headaches, abdominal pain, back pain or other physical symptoms that persist.

▶ Sleep problems. These may include insomnia, waking during the night or sleeping more than usual.

▶ Cognitive problems. You may have trouble concentrating, remembering things or making decisions.

▶ Thoughts of harming yourself or others. This may include thoughts of suicide or lashing out at others, including loved ones.

Treating depression

When it comes to mental health, medicine — as well as popular opinion — has made great strides in recent decades. Gone are the days when depression was considered an imagined problem or personality flaw. Depression is now recognized as the very real medical condition it is, and researchers have discovered several effective ways to treat it successfully — from medications and therapy to lifestyle changes.

Depression related to menopause is treated in the same way as depression during any other time of life. The treatment that's right for you will depend on personal factors, such as the severity of depression you're experiencing. Some people with mild cases of depression benefit from therapy alone. Others, with moderate to severe depression, find antidepressants to be necessary.

Your health care provider can help you find the right treatment or combination of treatments to help you not only cope — but live a healthy, active and full life.

ANTIDEPRESSANTS Many menopausal women find that taking a prescription medication is an effective way to manage their depression. Antidepressants are the most commonly prescribed medications for depression around the time of menopause.

Antidepressants are exactly what they sound like — medications that work against depression. Antidepressants go to work in your brain,

Depression: When should you seek help?

If you're experiencing any of the signs and symptoms of depression during menopause (or at any time), make an appointment with your health care provider.

Depression can range from feeling "blue" and not your usual self to deep feelings of hopelessness and despair. Even if you just wonder if you have depression, seeking professional help is always the right choice.

Don't let embarrassment or pride convince you to manage the condition on your own. Depression can get worse if it isn't treated, and can lead to other mental and physical health problems. The earlier you start treatment, the sooner you'll feel like yourself again.

If you're having suicidal thoughts, reach out to a trusted friend or family member, a leader in your faith community, or your health care provider. Or call a suicide hotline number to reach a trained counselor. (The National Suicide Prevention Lifeline, at 800-273-8255, is available to U.S. residents.) Suicide hotlines often offer anonymous, 24-hour help.

helping to stabilize chemicals called neurotransmitters that are involved in regulating mood.

There is no good or bad antidepressant — or one that will be a cure-all. The type of medication you should take, if any, depends on your situation. The length of time you will take antidepressants differs, too. When you start taking an antidepressant, it often takes three to four weeks to notice a change in your mood.

Lifestyle strategies for treating depression

Medications and professional counseling are often important, even vital, components of treating depression. But there are things you can do on your own, too. Try these actions for managing depression while continuing your other treatments.

▶ **Get enough sleep.** Practice good sleep hygiene to help you get enough, and regular, sleep. For sleep tips, see Chapter 6.

▶ **Exercise.** Try to get at least 30 minutes of physical activity on most days of the week. For best results, aim to exercise at a moderate intensity. (How do you know if you're exercising at moderate intensity? You should be able to talk, but not sing a song, during exercise.)

▶ **Take time for yourself.** Take a break from your daily stresses by spending some quiet time, every day, by yourself. Take a bath, read a book, go for a walk, or try some of the relaxation activities on page 91.

▶ **Keep the lines of communication open.** Talk to your family and friends about your feelings, or find a support group of women who are going through the same thing you're going through. Talking about your problems and challenges can help you manage them and put them in perspective

Try to be patient. It can take some time to find the right medication and dose for your situation. Sometimes you need to try two or three different medications or combinations to find the right fit. Stick with the program and work with your health care provider to find what works for you. It's worth it.

Once you start feeling better, it can be tempting to feel like you're "cured" and want to quit taking your medication. But antidepressants must be taken on a regular, consistent schedule to be effective. You should only stop under the advice of your health care provider. When it's time to discontinue your antidepressant, your health care provider may recommend that you wean off gradually to avoid withdrawal symptoms. In some cases, your health care provider may recommend you continue taking antidepressants indefinitely.

HORMONE THERAPY For some women, hormone therapy may be enough to treat mild mood problems at menopause. This is because hormone therapy can help reduce the menopausal symptoms, such as hot flashes and night sweats, that contribute to irritability, melancholy and depressive moods. Research also suggests that hormone therapy may help alleviate mild depression in menopausal women who aren't experiencing these symptoms, by helping to stabilize fluctuating hormones.

Depending on your symptoms and their severity, your health care provider might recommend trying hormone therapy — especially if you're also experiencing significant menopause symptoms. However, hormone therapy is not a replacement for antidepressants in women who have been diagnosed with moderate to severe depression. For more information on hormone therapy, see Chapter 10.

COGNITIVE BEHAVIORAL THERAPY The thoughts you have during depression can be painful and defeating. You may feel worthless and insignificant, or even just hollow or empty inside. These can be scary feelings, especially if you keep them bottled up.

That's where cognitive behavioral therapy (CBT) comes in. This form of therapy can help you improve these negative thoughts and feelings, and get you back on the road to good mental health. In CBT, a professional therapist helps you change your negative way of thinking — and the negative behaviors that often occur as a result.

Cognitive behavioral therapy is more than the opportunity to share what's on your mind. The process is action oriented and collaborative. Your therapist uses your sessions to help you identify the relationships between your thoughts, feelings and behaviors — then helps you set goals, and gives you the tools necessary to make changes in order to meet those goals. Your therapist may even ask you to keep a journal, write down behavior patterns or do other take-home work between appointments. The objective is to work together to change your thought processes, stop damaging behavior and recover from your depression.

Let's talk about stress

Stress — that pulse-quickening, muscle-tensing, adrenaline-releasing jolt you get during times of change or challenge — often gets a bad rap. But stress isn't always bad. In fact, in some situations, it can be quite helpful.

Stress, which is your brain's response to a change or demand, can help you take action, cause you to be more alert and give you energy when faced with danger. When you feel stress, your body responds by increasing (or, sometimes, decreasing) the release of certain "stress hormones" that help you manage and adapt to whatever it is that's causing your stress. It can be a great resource when you're faced with a quick-thinking situation, such as dodging out of the way of an oncoming car, or catching a child who is about to fall down a staircase.

But when you experience stress over the long term, it can harm both your mental and physical health. Instead of being helpful, that constant surge of stress hormones can negatively affect your body systems.

There are many reasons you may experience long-term stress during menopause. In addition to the myriad changes you're experiencing in your body, midlife can also be a time of changes in family, work and relationships. Combine hot flashes, aging parents, an empty nest (or a testy teen), retirement planning, fatigue and hormone fluctuations, and you have a combination strong enough to stress out even the most centered woman.

Some signs of stress are obvious — you can see or feel them. You may have headaches, stomachaches or trouble sleeping. You may tense your shoulders, clench your hands or tighten your jaw, often without even realizing it. You may jump to anger and irritability more quickly, feel down, and contract viruses — such as the flu or a cold — more frequently.

Other signs of stress are happening under the surface — with your hormones. Those hormone surges that are great for fight-or-flight situations can also cause your blood pressure, heart rate and blood sugar levels to rise. They may disrupt your menstrual cycle if you're still having your period, cause problems with your digestion, and even affect your immune system. The strain on your body from long-term stress can contribute to heart disease, high blood pressure, obesity, mental health disorders, diabetes and even skin problems, such as acne.

Signs and symptoms of stress to watch for include:

▶ A change in diet. You may eat less or more than you traditionally have.

▶ Memory loss. You may become forgetful, easily distracted and lack focus.

- A "short fuse." Your temper may flare unpredictably.

- Sleeping problems. You may have trouble falling asleep or trouble falling back asleep after waking at night.

- Control issues. You may worry that you have no control — or feel the need to exert too much control.

- Aches and pains. You may experience physical signs of stress, including headache, upset stomach, back pain, and just general aches and pains.

- Problems with motivation. You may have trouble completing tasks due to a lack of energy or drive.

With all of the responsibilities, obligations and concerns that a menopausal woman faces, it may seem impossible to get a grip on your stress. But it's not. There are many proven methods that will not only help you manage stress — but help you live a calmer, happier life in the process.

Managing stress

When you manage stress well, you can prevent it from becoming a significant issue in your life. Start by recognizing your triggers. Once you do this, it's easier to avoid, or manage, situations that cause you stress.

A good first step is to write down the activities or obligations that are stressful to you. Then, write down possible solutions. For instance, if being late to appointments causes you stress, decide to leave 10 minutes earlier than usual. Or if you feel there are too many demands on your time, take a critical look at your commitments and decide what can go. Looking at your challenges, and coming up with solutions in a calm, strategic way, can help you feel more in control when stressors do arise.

Of course, not all stress can be avoided. And some times in your life — like the menopause years — can cause an increase in your stress levels. So if you're feeling stress creep into your life, consider these techniques to help you cope:

PRACTICE MINDFULNESS There are many ways you might describe that feeling you get when your thoughts jump or wander from topic to topic, and idea to idea: "Unfocused." "Distracted." And, of course, "stressed out."

Everyday ways to practice mindfulness

Keep these techniques in mind when trying to work mindfulness into your daily life:

FOCUS ON WHAT'S IN FRONT OF YOU Consciously practice being more aware of your daily activities. As you go about your day, take the time to really hear the sounds around you — your fingers on the keyboard, the wind blowing through the trees. Look at the familiar objects in your life — your coffee mug, your favorite pair of shoes — with fresh eyes. See if you can notice new details in them.

It would be impossible to maintain complete focus all day long. Instead, set aside time each day to pay attention to what you're doing in the moment. If you're talking to a family member or co-worker, for instance, focus on what he or she is saying instead of letting your mind wander, or planning what you'll say next. If you're writing a to-do list, focus on the items you are writing, the feel of the pencil in your fingers, the texture and color of the paper you are writing on. If you find your mind wandering, gently return your focus to the present moment.

Our world is full of distractions that pull attention in multiple directions. You're in a conversation with a friend when the phone rings. You reach for your cellphone, and notice that you just got an email from your boss. Meanwhile, a screen pops up on your computer reminding you of that 2 p.m. meeting you scheduled yesterday. You remember you have to pick up bread before dinner, and — oh, yeah — you also need to pick up that prescription and a gift for your niece's birthday.

It's no wonder you may feel overwhelmed, anxious or just plain stressed out. It's hard to focus on the moment when there are so many things happening at any one time.

That's where mindfulness exercises come in. Mindfulness is setting aside these distractions and worries, and being fully present and aware in the moment. It's a way to focus on what is happening in front of you. See above for some suggestions on getting started.

The benefits of mindfulness are convincing. Practicing mindfulness can help reduce your stress and anxiety, manage depression, improve mood, and even help you cope with illness. It can help you relax and manage the demands on your life.

MEDITATE ON YOUR LOVED ONES Once a day, in a quiet moment, close your eyes and think of a person who is important to you. Then, remember specific details about this person. Picture this person's face. Hear the sound of his or her voice. Think about how you feel when you are with this person. Do this for two or three people in a row.

PRACTICE GRATITUDE It's easy to take the positive aspects of your life for granted. Be more aware of your good fortune by practicing gratitude. Each morning before you get out of bed, think about three things that make you feel grateful. These may be as simple as a sunny morning or getting an unexpected phone call from a friend.

DINE DELIBERATELY If you're like many women, when you sit down for a meal, you are often multitasking — watching TV, checking social media on your phone, maybe even working at your desk. Instead, avoid distractions while eating and focus on each bite of food. Notice how it looks. Notice its taste, and how it feels in your mouth as you chew it. This simple act of being present with your food can help refresh your mind.

RELAXATION THERAPIES It's been one of those days. You missed a deadline at work. Your teenager left the car in the driveway with an empty gas tank. Again. And in a particularly weak moment over lunch, you volunteered to throw a 50th birthday party for a friend … this Friday.

It's enough to stress anyone out. Fortunately, when it comes to managing stress, there are some specific relaxation techniques that have been proven to be effective. Try the following to manage your stress — and to help keep future stress at bay.

Take some deep breaths You can practice relaxation breathing almost anywhere — at your desk, in your living room just before the dinner rush or even in bed at night before you fall asleep. The key is finding a quiet, comfortable place where you can relax and focus for a few minutes. Then, close your eyes, and with one hand resting gently on your abdomen, breathe slowly and evenly — in through your nose, and out through your mouth.

As you focus on your breath, let other thoughts fall away. Focus your mind on the air passing in and out of your body, and the way your abdomen expands and falls with each breath. Feel your abdomen pushing your hand out as you fill your lungs, and letting it sink back as you fully exhale.

Continue this deep breathing for several minutes. If your mind starts to drift, don't worry. This is common. Just gently redirect it back to your breathing. Practice this breathing exercise throughout the day to help you relax, focus your energy and reduce stress.

Pay attention to your muscles Of all the physical side effects of stress, tense muscles are often the most apparent. Stress can cause you to tighten your shoulders, stiffen your neck, clench your hands, tighten your jaw muscles or grind your teeth — even when you're sleeping. In fact, often-times, you don't even realize you're doing these things until you feel those knots in your shoulders, the soreness in your jaw or that tension headache creep up the base of your neck.

There are a couple of ways you can help yourself feel less tense. Flexibility exercises, such as routine stretches or yoga, can help you relax your muscles and your mind. Massage also can be a powerful tension reducer. Neck, shoulder and upper back massages target the common culprits, but hand, face and foot massages also can be relaxing.

Treat yourself With so many demands on your time, it's easy to put yourself last. But taking the time to do things you enjoy can be a powerful and healthy way to combat stress. Each day, carve out time to focus on activities that are meaningful to you — perhaps reading a book, going for a walk, or playing or listening to music.

Practice stress-reducing exercises Quiet and gentle exercise programs, such as yoga and tai chi, can be a great way to de-stress. In particular, you may want to consider classes that include a meditation component.

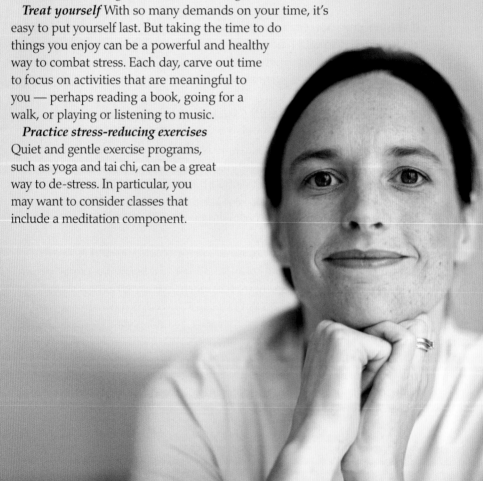

Stress management techniques

In addition to relaxation and mindfulness techniques, the following practices can help you live a healthier and less stressful life:

PRIORITIZE YOUR TIME It's easy to get bogged down in busy work, or tied to activities you don't particularly enjoy. Change this by taking a critical look at what's most important to you. Is it spending time with family? Making time for friends? Working on a hobby? Make conscious decisions about how you're going to spend your time, then carve out space in your week for those activities.

SAY NO Many women feel the need to "do it all." They want to be the perfect partner, mother, employee, friend, neighbor and volunteer. But when you try to do it all, someone usually suffers. And that someone is often you. Only take on commitments that you can manage — and that leaves time for your own interests and downtime. Saying no can be freeing.

SLEEP You've heard of beauty sleep — but getting a good night's sleep doesn't only help with the bags under your eyes. Being well-rested also helps promote mental health. It can help you think more clearly and prepare you to take on the challenges ahead.

ENERGIZE THE RIGHT WAY When stress leaves you feeling fatigued and weary, it's tempting to compensate with caffeine or high-sugar snack foods. But that short-term energy jolt will wear off, and you could wind up feeling more tired than you did before. Instead, fuel up with a healthy diet including fruits, vegetables, legumes and whole grains. And get plenty of physical activity. Exercise doesn't only help increase your energy, but can also relax your tense muscles and improve your mood.

TALK IT OUT Keeping your stress bottled up can make you feel worse. Talk to family or friends about the things that cause stress in your life. Sometimes just talking about it will make you feel better. If you're still feeling overwhelmed, considering talking to a professional. A counselor or therapist can help you find ways to better manage your stress.

AVOID UNHEALTHY COPING STRATEGIES It can be tempting to manage stress with unhealthy, short-term fixes, such as alcohol, drugs, tobacco or food. But healthier coping strategies — relaxation techniques, mindfulness practices or exercise — are always better options.

CHAPTER SIX

When you can't sleep

What you would give to enjoy a good night's sleep again. Remember back to your teens and early 20s when you could fall asleep the minute your head hit the pillow, and you would sleep so soundly that you barely moved. Those nights seem like a faded dream. Nowadays, sleep is often a struggle. You may have trouble falling asleep. During the night, you may toss and turn and wake up several times and find it hard to get back to sleep. In the morning, you may find yourself up with the birds, despite having a restless night. And because you aren't sleeping well, you may feel fatigued during the daytime.

As with other changes taking place in your life, it's easy to blame your sleep problems on menopause. But the truth is, your hormones are only partly to blame. There's no doubt that menopause can make getting a good night's sleep more difficult. But menopause is just one piece of a larger puzzle. Many factors affect your ability to sleep. As you age, your body and your life circumstances change. The cumulative effect of these changes is what often makes sleep more elusive in the second half of your life.

The good news is you don't have to live with poor sleep, spending your days feeling tired and unmotivated. Conditions such as insomnia, sleep apnea and Willis-Ekbom disease (formerly known as restless legs syndrome) can be treated. By understanding the changes happening in your life and how these changes may be affecting your sleep, you can take steps to help ensure that you get a good night's rest.

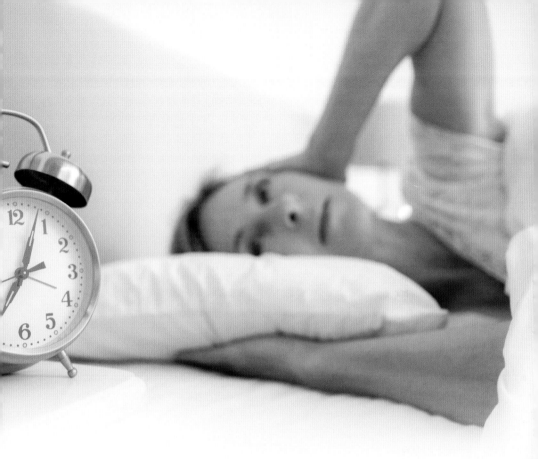

Normal sleep patterns

As you've likely learned over the years, not all sleep is the same. When you close your eyes and drift off into unconsciousness, your sleep follows a type of biological rhythm — a recurring sleep pattern known as the sleep-wake cycle.

Your sleep-wake cycle is influenced by your body's natural circadian rhythms. Circadian rhythms are cyclical changes — such as fluctuations in body temperature and hormone levels — driven by your brain's biological clock. The circadian system is highly influenced by day and night. Your natural circadian rhythms attempt to keep you awake during the daylight hours, and they prompt you to sleep once it becomes dark.

While most people's sleep-wake cycle follows a similar pattern, sleep needs and routines vary. Some people need more sleep, and others need less. Some people are morning people while others are night owls. Some people fall asleep the minute they get into bed while others need to read or listen to music to coax their brains to sleep.

Sleep patterns also vary with age. Between the ages of 50 and 60, sleep tends to become more restless and less refreshing. This is because more of your night is spent in light sleep and less of it in deep and dreaming sleep. In other words, your sleep-wake cycle is changing.

SLEEP CYCLES Sleep researchers have identified several stages of sleep that make up the sleep-wake cycle. These stages are divided into two main categories:

▶ **NREM sleep.** NREM stands for non-rapid eye movement. NREM consists of three stages of sleep, each deeper than the last.

Sleep stages

While you sleep, you move through a cycle of sleep stages. It takes about 90 to 110 minutes to complete a cycle, which is repeated approximately four to six times a night. Restful, restorative sleep occurs when you have the right balance of stages.

NREM sleep

N1 stage: Transitional sleep	During this stage, which lasts about five minutes, you transition from being awake to falling asleep. Your eyes move slowly behind your eyelids, and your brain waves and muscle activity slow down.
N2 stage: Light sleep	This is the first stage of true sleep. Your eye movement stops, your heart rate slows, and your body temperature decreases.
N3 stage: Deep sleep	In this stage of sleep, your brain waves are extremely slow, your blood pressure drops, and your breathing slows. During deep sleep, you're difficult to awaken, and if you are awakened, it takes you awhile to adjust.

REM sleep

Dreaming sleep	Following deep sleep, you enter REM sleep, where the majority of dreaming occurs. Your eyes move rapidly beneath your eyelids, your breathing is shallow, and your heart rate and blood pressure increase. During this stage, your arm and leg muscles become temporarily paralyzed.

▶ **REM sleep.** REM refers to rapid eye movement. In REM sleep, your eyes actually move back and forth. This is the stage of sleep when the majority of dreaming occurs.

Your nightly sleep journey begins in the first stage of NREM sleep, called N1, or transitional sleep, and it progresses to the next levels of NREM sleep before crossing over into REM sleep. This pattern repeats itself several times during the night.

Adults, on average, spend more than half of their total daily sleep time in N2 sleep, about 20 percent in REM sleep and the remaining time in other stages, mainly N3 sleep. However, with age, the amount of time spent in deep sleep and dream sleep decreases and lighter sleep increases.

So, if it seems that you just don't sleep like you used to, you're right. Beginning in your young adult and middle adult years, your sleep gradually becomes less sound. You experience more awakenings each night, and you're more aware of being awake.

HOURS OF SLEEP Do sleep patterns change because you simply need less sleep as you get older? There's no cut and dried answer. For the most part, studies suggest that older adults require just as much sleep as younger adults do. The recommended amount is at least seven hours a night.

There is some evidence that with age, both too much and too little sleep may be harmful to your health. A study showed that sleeping less than five hours a night or over nine hours a night may be associated with increased risk of heart disease or stroke. Other studies have shown that cognitive efficiency or mental sharpness is improved in adults who sleep six to eight hours a night as compared with those who sleep less or more.

What happens during menopause

If you're frustrated because you aren't sleeping well, you certainly aren't alone. A survey by the National Sleep Foundation found that almost half the American women age 40 and older have problems sleeping. The survey coincides with other studies indicating that the closer women get to menopause, the more sleep troubles they experience. Common complaints include difficulty falling asleep, waking up in the middle of the night and awakening early in the morning. It may not be surprising to you that poor sleep is often second only to hot flashes as the most common complaint of women going through the menopausal transition.

Interestingly, there are very few studies that have objectively examined sleep disorders in menopausal women. And of those that have been done, results have often differed. While some studies point to declining hormone levels as the reason you're not sleeping well, others suggest hormones play only a small role, if any. They conclude other symptoms or conditions are interfering with your sleep, or that your problems have nothing to do with menopause at all; rather, they're a reflection of natural aging or significant changes taking place in your life. In addition, there's some evidence that how well you slept in your younger years may be a precursor to how well you'll sleep in your later years.

REDUCED HORMONES As you've learned in previous chapters, beginning at around age 40 — although it can happen later — your ovaries gradually begin producing decreased amounts of estrogen and progesterone. These hormones have a wide range of effects, including interaction with specific brain chemicals (neurotransmitters) that help promote sleep. So it makes sense that as hormone production gradually declines, the simple act of falling asleep and staying asleep may become more difficult.

RELATED CONDITIONS Other studies suggest that it's not specifically the decline in hormone levels that impact sleep during menopause, but other conditions that often result from the hormonal changes.

A good example is hot flashes. If you've experienced hot flashes, you know the nighttime disruption they can cause. As explained in Chapter 4, hot flashes result from declining estrogen levels and changes in your body's internal thermostat. Hot flashes and night sweats may leave you hot and sweating one moment and cold and shivering the next, making it tough to sleep. Some women even need to get up from bed and change their clothes after a particularly drenching episode. If you're among the many women who struggle with hot flashes, your inability to get a good night's sleep is intricately tied to the hot and cold routine you dance to each night.

Other conditions that are more prevalent during menopause and that also can interfere with sleep are sleep apnea and restless legs syndrome (Willis-Ekbom disease). At least one study found that more than half the women who complained of trouble sleeping during menopause had sleep apnea, restless legs or both.

NATURAL AGING Some research suggests that hormones have nothing to do with poor sleep. These studies conclude that sleep efficiency naturally deteriorates over time, meaning that loss of sleep is more likely to be an effect of natural aging than of declining hormones. Another possibility is an intermingling of the two — your age and your hormones are both working against you.

LIFE CIRCUMSTANCES What doctors and researchers are finding is that as women transition through midlife, there's often a lot going on in their lives. In addition to changing hormones and natural aging, they're dealing with life circumstances. Midlife is when a variety of changes can occur, some of them significant. Often, these changes produce stress, which in turn can interfere with your ability to sleep. When you're experiencing menopause, it's easy to blame everything on your hormones — or lack of them. But is that the true cause?

Stressful events Like many women in midlife, you may find yourself dealing with significant life challenges. Examples include job-related issues, loss of life partners through divorce or death, children moving away, and caregiving for elderly parents. During the day when you're busy, you may be able to keep the stress at bay. But at night, when you try to rest and relax, the worry and anxiety come to the foreground, affecting your ability to sleep.

Changing routines You may find that as you get older you're less physically or socially active than you once were. A lack of activity can interfere with a good night's sleep. Also, the less active you are, the more likely you may be to take a nap during the day, making it more difficult to sleep at night.

Health issues Midlife is often when medical conditions develop that can interfere with sleep, such as back problems, arthritis or thyroid issues. You may begin experiencing bladder problems and find yourself waking up at night to go to the bathroom. In addition, the older you get, the more likely you are to take medications. Some medications can interfere with sleep. Common medications that can affect sleep are bronchodilators, steroids, thyroid hormones and certain antidepressants.

SLEEP HISTORY Has sleep always been a problem for you? A recent study suggests that your ability to sleep during your younger years may be predictive of how well you sleep in later years. Researchers at the University of Pennsylvania found that women in their late 30s and into their 40s who had trouble sleeping were more than three times more likely to experience sleep difficulties during menopause than were women of the same age who had an easier time sleeping when they were younger. The study also found that women who had sleep problems prior to menopause and who experienced hot flashes during menopause were the most likely to encounter sleep troubles.

The next step

The key message here is that often times it's not just one factor that's making sleep difficult as you enter menopause but a number of issues converging together. The bigger question, of course, is what can you do about it?

The first step is to try and peel back the layers to determine the source of the unrest. Is it stress? Is it hormones? Is it a combination of several things? If your sleep troubles are moderate to severe, you may need the help of your health care provider to help decipher the possible causes and determine potential treatments.

A number of options exist to treat menopause-related insomnia. For milder symptoms, a few changes to your daily and nightly routines may do the trick. For more-severe symptoms, behavioral therapy or medications may be necessary. If your difficult nights are a result of sleep apnea or restless legs syndrome, those conditions can be successfully treated as well.

Overcoming insomnia

If you have difficulty falling asleep, staying asleep or both, you have insomnia. With insomnia, you may wake up feeling groggy and unrefreshed, which can take a toll on your ability to function during the day. Insomnia can sap not only your energy level and your mood but also affect your health, work performance and quality of life.

For insomnia that occurs during menopause, your health care provider may ask a number of questions, and you may even be asked to take part in a sleep study to determine if there's a specific cause for the problem. For example, what you think is insomnia may actually be sleep apnea. Once a diagnosis of insomnia is made, you and your doctor can determine the best form of treatment. A variety of therapies exist to help improve sleep. Sometimes just a few changes to your sleep routine is all you need (see pages 100-101).

BEHAVIORAL THERAPY As with so many other aspects of your life, your habits are important. Good sleep habits help promote sound sleep. Behavioral therapy is about teaching you good sleep behaviors and specific strategies to improve your sleep. Behavioral therapy is generally taught by a sleep specialist, and it's often equally or more effective than sleep medications.

There are several components to behavioral therapy for sleep:

Sleep education Often, the first step in behavioral therapy is learning what may be hampering your sleep and what actions you can take to improve your sleep. Good sleep habits include having a regular sleep schedule, avoiding stimulating activities before bed and creating a comfortable sleep environment.

Relaxation techniques These help you control your breathing, heart rate, muscle tension and mood so that you can relax and fall asleep. Techniques used to help promote sleep include progressive muscle relaxation, biofeedback and deep breathing exercises. A sleep specialist can teach you how to perform these techniques.

Sleep restriction With this form of treatment, you decrease the amount of time you spend in bed, causing partial sleep deprivation, which makes it easier to fall asleep the next night. Once your sleep has improved, your time in bed is gradually increased.

Stimulus control This therapy is aimed at reducing your worry and anxiety about being able to fall sleep. Rather than forcing yourself to sleep, you do something relaxing that you enjoy until you're sleepy. Once you go to bed, if you aren't asleep within a few minutes, you get out of bed and read or listen to soothing music until you're sleepy again — eating or using an electronic device isn't allowed.

Cognitive therapy Cognitive therapy involves taking action before bed to help control or eliminate negative thoughts and worries that keep you awake. You might write down your worries in a journal or practice a relaxation technique such as meditation. This therapy also involves eliminating false or worrisome beliefs about sleep, such as the idea that a single restless night will make you sick or ruin the next day.

PRESCRIPTION MEDICATIONS Sometimes a change in sleeping habits may not be enough. Or it may take awhile for you to master various behavioral techniques. The next option is usually medication. In general, long-term use of prescription medications to promote sleep isn't recommended because the medications can produce side effects and some may be habit forming. However, medications may be used on a short-term basis to help you through an especially rocky period. A number of different options exist.

Hormone therapy Hormone therapy is the most effective treatment for relieving menopausal symptoms. If your sleep difficulties are severe and accompanied by other menopausal symptoms, such as hot flashes, your health care provider may recommend hormone therapy in the lowest dose needed to provide symptom relief. Whether you're a candidate for hormone

10 steps to better sleep

You might not be able to control all of the factors that interfere with your sleep, but you can adopt habits that encourage better sleep.

▶ **Forgo naps.** Naps can make it more difficult to fall asleep at night. If you can't get by without a nap, limit it to no more than 30 minutes and don't nap after 3 p.m.

▶ **Check your medications.** Talk to your health care provider or pharmacist to see if any medications you're taking may be contributing to your insomnia. Also check the labels of nonprescription products to see if they contain caffeine or other stimulants, such as pseudoephedrine.

▶ **Exercise and stay active.** Activity helps promote a good night's sleep. Get at least 30 minutes of vigorous exercise each day, but make sure you do so at least five to six hours before bedtime. Exercising too close to bedtime will keep you awake.

▶ **Avoid or limit caffeine and alcohol.** Caffeine and alcohol can make it more difficult to achieve sound sleep. Make it a point not to have any caffeine after lunchtime. Besides coffee, caffeine is found in tea, energy drinks, some sodas and chocolate. Also limit or avoid alcohol in the evening. Initially, alcohol may make you sleepy, but it also causes you to awaken during the night.

▶ **Keep your bedtime snack small.** Eating too much late in the evening can cause stomach upset and digestion problems that keep you awake. Also don't drink too much fluid before bed, or you will wake to use the bathroom during the night.

▶ **Relax before bed.** Try to put your worries and concerns aside when you get into bed. Even better, plan a time during the early part of the day to address your worries, so they don't weigh on you when it's time to sleep. Create a relaxing bedtime ritual. A warm bath before bedtime can help prepare you for sleep. Other options include reading a book, breathing exercises, yoga or prayer. Don't bring TVs, computers, your cellphone or other screens into your bedroom. The light can interfere with your sleep-wake cycle and the stimulation can prevent you from falling asleep. Remember, your bedroom is only for sleep and sex!

▶ **Make your bedroom comfortable.** Close your bedroom door or create a subtle background noise, such as a running fan, to help drown out other noises. Keep your bedroom temperature comfortable — make sure it's not too warm, especially if you're experiencing hot flashes.

▶ **Stick to a schedule.** Keep your bedtime and wake time consistent from day to day, including on weekends.

▶ **Hide the clocks.** Set your alarm so that you know when to get up, but then hide all clocks in your bedroom, including your cellphone, so you don't worry about what time it is if you wake up.

▶ **Don't 'try' to sleep.** The harder you try, the more awake you'll become. If you can't fall asleep, get out of bed and read or listen to soothing music in another room until you become drowsy, then go back to bed.

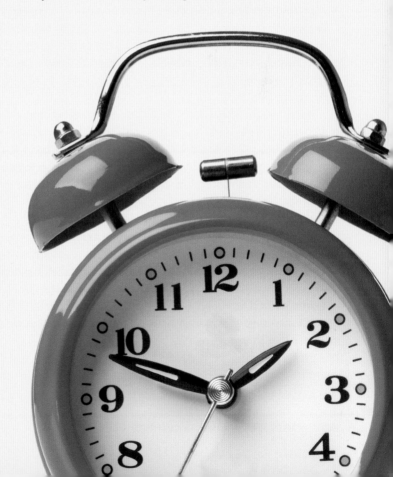

therapy will also depend on your personal and family medical history. Hormone therapy isn't recommended long term because of potential risks. For more on hormone therapy, see Chapter 10.

Sedatives and hypnotics Sleeping pills may be prescribed for a short period, such as a couple of weeks, to help break a cycle of insomnia.

▶ **Short-acting nonbenzodiazepines.** These medications include the drugs eszopiclone (Lunesta), zaleplon (Sonata) and zolpidem (Ambien). The medications act on brain receptors to slow down your nervous system. They may help you fall asleep, and the long-acting medications can help you stay asleep.

▶ **Benzodiazepines.** They include the older medications clonazepam (Klonopin), diazepam (Valium) and lorazepam (Ativan). Benzodiaze-pines can help you both fall asleep and stay asleep, but they may have significant side effects, such as next day drowsiness, and they can lead to dependence.

▶ **Melatonin agonist.** The medication ramelteon (Rozerem) works like the natural hormone melatonin produced by your body, helping to regulate your sleep-wake cycle (circadian rhythm). Some small trials have found ramelteon beneficial in helping people fall asleep more quickly and slightly increasing their total sleep time.

Antidepressants The drug doxepin (Silenor) has been approved for the treatment of chronic insomnia. Other antidepressants that may be prescribed to help promote sleep because of their sedating effects include amitriptyline, mirtazapine (Remeron) and trazodone. Sedating antidepressants taken in low doses aren't habit-forming, and they can be used for a longer period than other sleep medications.

OTHER TREATMENTS Like many women, you may prefer help for your sleep troubles that doesn't involve the use of medication. Here are some alternative therapies that may be worth a try. The therapies are likely to be more effective if your sleep problems are related to stress.

Acupuncture During an acupuncture session, a practitioner places many thin needles in your skin at specific points on your body. There's some evidence that this practice may be beneficial for people with insomnia; however, more research is needed. If you choose to try acupuncture, ask your health care provider how to find a qualified practitioner.

Beware of nonprescription sleep aids

There are several over-the-counter products designed to help you sleep. But just because they're available without a prescription doesn't mean you should take them. In general, over-the-counter sleep aids aren't recommended for long-term use, and many aren't regulated by the FDA.

▶ **Diphenhydramine.** Many over-the-counter sleep products contain diphenhydramine, a sedating antihistamine. Antihistamines may initially make you groggy, but they can reduce the quality of your sleep and can cause daytime sleepiness, dizziness, blurred vision and dry mouth. Antihistamines can also worsen urinary problems.

▶ **Melatonin.** Melatonin is a hormone that's secreted by the brain's pineal gland to help control your natural sleep-wake cycle. The hormone is sold as a supplement and marketed as a treatment for insomnia. While a few studies have shown it to be helpful, no convincing evidence exists to prove that melatonin is an effective treatment for menopause-related sleep disorders. The supplement is generally considered safe when taken for less than three months. Side effects can include headache and daytime sleepiness.

▶ **Valerian.** Supplements made from this plant are sometimes taken as sleep aids. Although a few studies indicate some therapeutic benefit, other studies haven't produced the same results. Valerian generally doesn't appear to cause side effects. However, if taken in high doses or used long term, it could possibly lead to liver problems.

Yoga Some studies suggest that performing yoga regularly can improve your sleep. Plus, the risks are limited. It might be worth it to give yoga a try and see if it helps you to relax and rest. Be sure to start slow and work with an instructor who listens to you and helps adapt poses to your needs and limitations.

Meditation There's evidence that meditation also may improve sleep in some individuals by promoting relaxation and reducing anxiety. Like yoga, it may be worth experimenting with this relaxation technique to see if it might alleviate your restless nights. Again, seek out a qualified instructor. Other positive health effects from regular meditation include reduced stress and reduced blood pressure.

THE BOTTOM LINE You may find that you need to experiment with a couple of different approaches to find a combination that works for you. The most important first step is to talk to your health care provider and discuss what strategies might work best. You also need to be patient. It often takes a few weeks for some treatments to become effective.

Treating sleep apnea

Insomnia is common in menopausal women, but for some, breathing problems may be behind the interrupted sleep. Studies show that after menopause, women are at increased risk of sleep apnea.

Sleep apnea is a potentially serious sleep disorder in which your breathing repeatedly stops and starts. The most common form of sleep apnea, obstructive sleep apnea, occurs when the tissues and muscles in the back of your throat relax. Your airway narrows or closes, and you can't take in an adequate breath. Your brain senses this inability to breathe and briefly rouses you from sleep so you can reopen your airway. The awakening is usually so brief that you don't remember it. The trouble is, this generally happens several times during the night. As a result, you aren't able to enter periods of deep and restful sleep.

Among women, sleep apnea is most common during and after menopause. In fact, after menopause, women develop sleep apnea at a rate similar to men. Most often, the reason is related to weight.

In both men and women, the strongest risk factor for obstructive sleep apnea is obesity. As you may already know, during and after menopause, women tend to gain weight. This includes weight gain in your neck, which can place pressure on your airway. Additionally, the hormonal changes associated with menopause increase your risk of developing sleep apnea.

For milder cases of sleep apnea, your health care provider may suggest lifestyle changes, such as losing weight, to improve your sleep. If your symptoms are moderate to severe, additional treatments are available.

DEVICES AND PROCEDURES There are a number of different products available to treat sleep apnea, but a lot of the over-the-counter devices are ineffective. The best way to treat sleep apnea is with a machine obtained from your health care provider.

Continuous positive airway pressure (CPAP) With this treatment, a machine delivers air pressure by way of soft prongs that go into the nostrils or a mask that's placed over your nose while you sleep. The air pressure is just enough to keep your upper airway passages open, preventing apnea. CPAP is the most common and most effective method of treating sleep apnea. Some people, however, find the device cumbersome or uncomfortable, and it takes awhile to adjust to wearing it. You may need to try more than one type of mask to find one that's comfortable. A humidifier attached to the CPAP system can help prevent a dry throat or stuffy nose. Check with your provider to see what comfort measures are available to help you adjust to using CPAP.

Strategies for overcoming sleep apnea

If your sleep apnea is very mild, you may be able to treat it on your own with some changes to your diet and daily routine. These strategies can improve your sleep:

▶ **Lose excess weight.** This step is key. Even a slight loss in weight may help improve sleep apnea. In some cases, returning to a healthy weight can resolve the problem entirely. If you need to lose weight, talk to your doctor about the best type of program for you and how to get started.

▶ **Exercise.** Each day, try to get at least 30 minutes of moderate activity, such as a brisk walk. Exercise may help ease obstructive sleep apnea symptoms by helping you lose weight.

▶ **Avoid alcohol and certain medications.** Alcohol and medications such as tranquilizers and sleeping pills relax the muscles in the back of your throat, interfering with breathing.

▶ **Don't sleep on your back.** Sleeping on your back can cause your tongue and soft palate to rest against the back of your throat and block your airway. To prevent sleeping on your back, try sewing a tennis ball in the back of your pajama top to keep you from rolling onto your back. Using a body pillow also can help keep you on your side when you sleep.

▶ **Keep your nasal passages open.** Use a saline nasal spray or nasal rinse before bed to help open your nasal passages, improving breathing. Don't use nasal decongestants or antihistamines without talking to your doctor. They're generally recommended only for short-term use.

Oral appliances Another option is to use an oral device that positions your lower jaw slightly forward, resulting in a more open airway. Some people find oral appliances to be easier and more comfortable than CPAP. However, the oral appliances may not be effective in everyone, and some patients develop changes in their bites with long-term use. A sleep specialist or qualified dentist can help determine if an oral appliance is right for you.

SURGERY Sleep apnea surgery is generally performed only in individuals with severe diseases who cannot tolerate CPAP. Surgery may also be recommended for those with certain jaw structure problems. The goal of surgery is to enlarge the airway by removing or tightening tissues and muscles that may block your upper air passages. These procedures may be combined with removal of enlarged tonsils or adenoids.

Dealing with restless legs

Willis-Ekbom disease, formerly known as restless legs syndrome, is a disorder that becomes more common with age. Although the condition hasn't been linked to menopause, a few studies suggest that it tends to occur more frequently in women experiencing hot flashes. For some women, part of the reason they have difficulty falling asleep at night is because their legs feel restless and uncomfortable.

People with Willis-Ekbom disease have an uncontrollable urge to move their legs during rest, often with unpleasant sensations in their legs or feet. Symptoms typically develop in the evening or at night while sitting or lying down. Often, getting up and walking will temporarily ease the unpleasant feelings, which are often described as crawling, creeping, antsy, pulling, throbbing, aching or itching.

WHAT YOU CAN DO Several prescription medications are available that may help reduce the restlessness in your legs. If your symptoms are severe, see your health care provider. You may also be tested for iron deficiency, which can be associated with restless legs symptoms.

Simple lifestyle changes also may help alleviate your symptoms. Here are some strategies to try:

Soak in a warm bath Soaking in a bath and massaging your legs in the evening can help relax your muscles and ease the restless symptoms.

Apply warm or cool packs Use of heat or cold, or alternating use of the two, may help lessen the uncomfortable sensations in your legs and feet.

Practice relaxation techniques, such as meditation or yoga Stress can aggravate restless legs symptoms. Experiment with different techniques and find a way to relax in the evening that works for you.

Establish good sleep hygiene Fatigue also tends to worsen symptoms. If you're overly tired, your symptoms are likely to be worse. Practice good sleep habits (see pages 100-101).

Exercise Get at least 30 minutes of moderate exercise most days of the week. Exercise helps prevent symptoms.

Avoid caffeine and alcohol Sometimes cutting back on caffeine improves symptoms. Avoid caffeine-containing products, including chocolate, coffee, tea and soft drinks, for a few weeks to see if this helps. Also see what happens if you eliminate alcohol. Alcohol is thought to aggravate symptoms in some individuals.

Stay positive

When you're tired and fatigued because you're not sleeping well, it's easy to feel down. You might feel as if you'll never sleep well again. That's not true; you will. Keep in mind that this is a phase in life you're going through. Also keep in mind that the journey doesn't have to be miserable. If a few adjustments to your evening and nighttime habits aren't helpful, talk to your health care provider. He or she can prescribe specific therapies or medication to help get your sleep back in sync so that you can get out and enjoy this new chapter in your life.

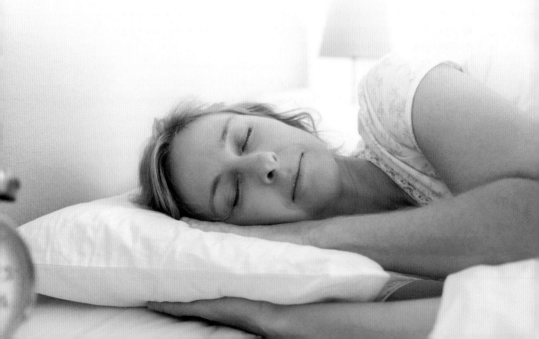

CHAPTER SEVEN

Changes in your sexual life and health

Menopause means you can no longer get pregnant. But that's no reason to stop having sex. Many women enjoy satisfying sex and intimacy well into old age.

You may face some challenges along the way. The transition to menopause may bring about changes in your sex drive, your vagina or your feelings about your own sex appeal. That's normal. There are plenty of lifestyle changes, bedroom tricks, drugstore gels and prescription medications that can help bring your sexy back.

Sex may be the last thing on your mind right now. If you've been with your partner for a long time, you may actually be grateful that the frequent, feverish trysts of your younger years have transformed into a cooler, easier companionship. Just remember that there's no time limit on feeling sexy or being sexual. Every long-lasting relationship can benefit from butterflies, longing, spontaneity, fun and physical closeness. Sex isn't the only thing that holds two people together, but it can help strengthen your connection.

Of course, women without partners aren't excused from this conversation either. Even if you're not having sex with a partner now, you may decide to engage in a sexual relationship at a later time. All women deserve to enjoy sex long after their last menstrual period, if they want to.

The myth of midlife chastity

It's rare to see older couples kissing, shedding their clothes, or having sex on TV or in the movies. Films that cast older couples — such as the 2003 romantic comedy hit *Something's Gotta Give*, starring 66-year-old Jack Nicholson and 57-year-old Diane Keaton — seem bold and striking, because this is such an unusual choice. Off-screen, real-life examples of a red-hot older sex life can be hard to come by, too. Many people grow up believing that their parents and grandparents aren't having sex. And few parents and grandparents go out of their way to publicly dispute this belief.

Given this dearth of role models for sex at midlife and beyond, many women believe that sex naturally ends at a certain point. When women start feeling old, due to the changes that manifest during menopause, they sometimes automatically assume they shouldn't be sexual anymore.

Nonsense. The notion that sex is over at 50 is a myth. Challenge this myth anytime it creeps into your head. The truth is that your parents and grandparents probably were (or are) having sex. People can (and do) have sex right up until they die. In fact, older women may be having sex a lot more than you think. In a recent study of more than 2,000 women, nearly 60 percent of those age 60 and older who were married or living with a partner were sexually active. That's the majority, not the minority! Further, 37 percent of women age 80 and older who had a romantic partner were sexually active.

Give yourself permission to be sexual well into your golden years. If you need help, talk to your health care provider, a counselor or a sex therapist.

Common sexual changes during menopause

While the belief that all older adults are celibate isn't true, there are some genuine changes that occur during menopause that can alter your sex life. For some women, sex is more enjoyable. Not having to worry about getting pregnant can be liberating and sexy. Some couples also become empty nesters around the time of menopause, and this can add to the sense of feeling uninhibited. When grown children move out, privacy and sexual spontaneity may return. Spur-of-the-moment sex on the couch becomes a real possibility again, even in the afternoon!

However, many women find that they think about sex less often or don't enjoy it as much after menopause. Many menopausal changes can contribute to these feelings: Decreasing estrogen levels can cause drier vaginal tissues and thinning of the vagina, resulting in painful or uncomfortable sex.

In addition, night sweats can disturb your sleep and make you feel too exhausted or sweaty for sex. Emotional changes can make you feel too stressed for sex. And weight gain can make you feel too insecure for sex.

How do you know if you have a problem? There's no magical number of times you should have sex or reach orgasm each week. The real key is whether sexual changes are troubling to you or your partner. If sexual changes associated with the menopausal transition bother you or cause strife in your relationship, that's a problem. It's time to focus on solutions.

Here's a summary of some of the most common sexual issues that occur at this time.

LOW SEX DRIVE (LOW LIBIDO) Fluctuations in your sex drive are a normal part of every relationship and every stage of life. It's common to feel revved up at the beginning of a new relationship or while on a romantic trip. On the flip side, your sex drive may drop after you have a baby or get bored with a relationship.

You should know that there are two types of sexual desire. One is spontaneous desire — this is the biological drive or craving for sex. With this type of desire, you may have a sexual thought after watching a steamy movie and want to initiate sex with your partner. The other type of desire is called receptive desire. In this type of desire, sex isn't on your mind, but the ingredients are in place for you to be willing when your partner initiates.

Spontaneous desire relies heavily on hormones, and it can plummet for some women as hormone levels shift during menopause. Men also experience a decrease in spontaneous desire with age, but it happens at a much slower rate — more like a slow leak.

If your spontaneous desire for sex declines, it can be difficult to recover. But you can make up for any loss in spontaneous desire by maximizing your receptive desire. How? Optimize all of the ingredients that contribute to your willingness to have sex. These ingredients differ among women and are different over time, but they usually fall into four general categories — biological issues, psychological issues, relationship issues and life issues.

Review the list on the next page and circle every issue that's impacting your willingness to be sexual. Add in extra factors of your own. Ask yourself: Which issues on this list jump out? What are the big things that are getting in the way of being sexual? Could I enjoy sexual activity if any of these barriers were removed? For example, could you let everything else go if you felt close to your partner again or if you didn't have pain during intercourse?

Create a plan to address your turnoffs and take full advantage of your receptive desire. When your spontaneous desire was kicking, this conscientious approach to sex probably wasn't necessary. But, now, it's essential to recalculate your desire equation. As part of your plan, meet with your health care provider to identify any health conditions or medications that may curb your desire.

Biological issues

Vaginal dryness

Sexual pain

Other chronic pain or arthritis

Other health concerns or illnesses

Incontinence

Sleep problems

Low energy or fatigue

Hot flashes

Weight gain

Medication side effects

Other: _____

Relationship issues

Unresolved relationship conflicts

Inadequate sexual stimulation

Partner's loss of interest in sex or sexual dysfunction

Partner's renewed interest in sex

Lack of emotional closeness or connectedness

Poor communication

Lack of privacy

Opposing schedules

Other: _____

Psychological issues

Anxiety

Depression

Stress

History of unwanted sexual experiences

Low self-esteem

Poor body image

Substance abuse

Other: _____

Life and socio-economic issues

Stress from caregiving

Work deadlines

Busy schedules

Limited sex education

Conflict with personal, family or religious values

Other: _____

Also, be sure to discuss your feelings with your partner, who may feel discouraged or slighted by your new lack of interest in sex. Low sex drive can be very difficult on your relationship. It's natural to feel frustrated or sad if you aren't able to be as sexy and romantic as you want — or used — to be. At the same time, low desire can make your partner feel rejected, which leads to conflicts and fighting. And this type of relationship turmoil can further reduce your desire for sex. Help your partner understand what you're feeling and identify how he or she can help.

Even if you're able to increase your receptive desire, your partner will need to initiate sex for you to be receptive. If this isn't your usual pattern, you may need to change things.

PROBLEMS WITH AROUSAL Like desire, arousal also can change with menopause. Arousal refers to your readiness for sex. During arousal, your breathing and heart rate speed up, your nipples become tingly and erect, and the blood flow to your genitals increases. This causes your labia, clitoris and upper vagina to swell in anticipation of sex.

For many women, all of these processes are thwarted during menopause. The decline in estrogen can cause vaginal dryness and reduced blood flow to the vulva, clitoris and vagina, causing arousal to take longer or be harder to achieve.

The sensations and pleasure that you typically experience during sex may change significantly. You may need more time for foreplay and more emphasis on strong clitoral stimulation before jumping into intercourse.

CHANGES IN ORGASM In addition to arousal struggles, there can be changes in orgasm. In particular, the clitoris — a key pleasure zone for most women — can become less sensitive. If you do reach orgasm, it may not be as long or intense as it used to be.

It can be frustrating if your usual lovemaking routine suddenly doesn't do it for you anymore. Take comfort in knowing that there's nothing wrong with you or your partner. This is a normal part of the menopausal transition. You can also consider it a license to experiment with new tricks and positions. In addition, you may benefit from vaginal lubricants and moisturizers as well as vibrators to provide extra stimulation. You'll learn more about these accessories on pages 120-122.

SEXUAL PAIN The medical term for painful intercourse is dyspareunia (dis-puh-ROO-nee-uh), which is defined as persistent or recurrent genital pain that occurs just before, during or after intercourse. Many women experience painful intercourse at some point in their lives. Treatments focus on the underlying cause of the pain and can help eliminate or reduce this common problem. (They'll be discussed in more detail later in this chapter.)

No matter how much you love your partner and want to be intimate, there's no reason to grin and bear painful intercourse. If you can't get relief on your own, seek help from your health care provider.

Vaginal dryness As you read in Chapter 3, insufficient lubrication is a very common, early sign of menopause. For some women, this early sign of menopause grows to be a severe, distressing problem. And dryness can cause significant discomfort and pain during initial penetration.

Vaginal dryness is commonly part of a larger condition known as genitourinary syndrome of menopause (GSM). As discussed on pages 59-60, in this condition, the vulvar skin becomes thin and dry. Ongoing burning, itching, irritation, and even spotting or bleeding also can occur. All of these signs and symptoms can dampen your desire or arousal and make sex painful.

Vaginal moisturizers and lubricants are often used as an initial treatment for these conditions. Vaginal estrogen or the oral medication ospemifene (Osphena) also may be used for moderate to severe cases of GSM. In addition, regular sexual activity or use of a vibrator may be recommended, if you can engage in these activities without pain. Regular sexual activity

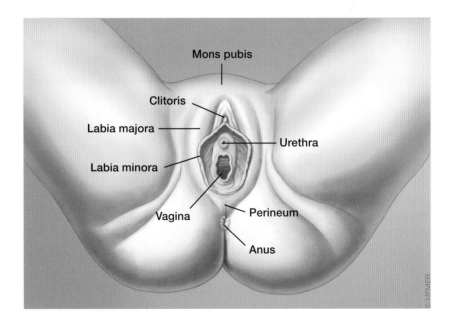

— including massage and oral stimulation — can help increase arousal and promote blood flow to the genital area, which can help rejuvenate the area.

Vulvodynia Chronic pain in the area around the opening of your vagina (vulva) with no observable, physical reason is called vulvodynia. The pain, burning, stinging or irritation associated with vulvodynia may be constant or occasional and can last for months to years. You may feel the pain in your entire vulvar area (generalized), or it may be localized to a certain area, such as the opening of your vagina (vestibule). The latter is called vestibulodynia. Symptoms can make you so uncomfortable that sitting for long periods is difficult and sex is unthinkable.

Special circumstances: Lesbian relationships

Navigating menopausal sex may be significantly harder for lesbian couples than heterosexual couples. Unless there's a big age difference, both women hit menopause at about the same time.

There are many experiences in life that are fun to share with your partner, but menopause isn't necessarily one of them. If you and your partner simultaneously experience menopausal symptoms — including trouble sleeping, irritability, weight gain and vaginal dryness — it can put a lot of stress on your relationship. Plus, you may both lose your spontaneous desire for sex at the same time as estrogen levels drop. So no one is initiating anything.

If you're in this situation, it's important for you and your partner to figure out how to maximize willingness for both of you. A high level of mutual willingness can help offset a loss of spontaneous desire. Review all of the issues that can undo your desire for sex (above), and work diligently to remove these barriers. Working with a counselor or sex therapist can help.

Treatment depends on the severity of symptoms but often starts with self-care measures. Try to avoid any vaginal irritants, including soaps, detergents, dryer sheets, moistened wipes, perfumes, douches, spermicides, scented toilet paper, bubble baths, and flavored or warming vaginal lubricants. Tightfitting pantyhose and nylon underwear also can be problematic, restricting airflow to your genital area and leading to increased moisture and irritation. Switch to white cotton underwear and consider sleeping with no underwear to promote ventilation and dryness. Clean the affected area with plain water and apply a preservative-free emollient, such as plain petroleum jelly, to create a protective barrier. Cold compresses or warm water baths also may help.

You may need vaginal lubricants and moisturizers to make sex more comfortable. Topical lidocaine may be another option. Your doctor may recommend applying this numbing medication before sexual activity or as needed for comfort. For moderate or severe cases that don't respond to these treatments, it may be necessary to consider topical or oral medications for chronic pain, pelvic floor physical therapy, or even surgery. Pain control takes time, sometimes three to six weeks. You may need to work with a gynecologist or women's health specialist to find the right mix of therapies for you.

Other conditions and surgeries Many other conditions and surgical side effects can cause sexual pain. Pain with initial penetration can be caused by a cut made during childbirth to enlarge the birth canal (episiotomy) or an infection in your genital area or urinary tract. Deep pain can be caused by scarring from pelvic surgery, including hysterectomy, or by treatments for cancer. In addition, many gynecological conditions can be to blame, including pelvic floor dysfunction. (See page 137.) Work with your health care provider to determine the cause of pain, so you can treat it accordingly.

Strategies for more-satisfying sex

No matter what sexual setbacks you face during menopause, there are many treatments out there for the taking. Your health care provider can guide you to the best solution for your particular situation, but there's little harm in trying a few measures on your own. Think of menopause as an opportunity to revive your sex life and your relationship.

SELF-CARE MEASURES If you have minor sexual symptoms, this is a good place to start. You can also use self-care measures to protect your sexual health, before symptoms begin.

Avoid products that irritate your vagina This is particularly important for vaginal dryness or irritation, but it's good advice all-around. As mentioned earlier, skip bubble baths, dryer sheets, moistened wipes, perfumes and other irritants. Remember that nylon underwear can be irritating, too. Find something sexy in 100 percent cotton.

Practice pelvic floor (Kegel) exercises These exercises can increase blood flow to your vagina and strengthen the muscles involved in orgasm. If you need help identifying your pelvic floor muscles, stop urination in midstream. But don't do Kegel exercises while you're urinating — only use this technique to isolate the correct muscles. Then, lie on your back and practice contracting the muscles for five seconds and then relaxing them for five seconds. Work up to keeping the muscles contracted for 10 seconds at a time, with 10 seconds in between. Repeat three times a day. Once you've got the technique down, you can do Kegel exercises discreetly just about anywhere.

Exercise Physical activity can increase your energy, lift your mood and help you feel good about your body.

Avoid smoking and alcohol Cigarette smoking can reduce blood flow to the vagina and contribute to vaginal dryness. Alcohol can slow down your biological sexual response. You may think that alcohol helps put you in the mood, but the result can be the opposite.

Adjust your attitude Remember that your brain is your most powerful sexual organ. Focus on your attitude and mindset about sex.

INTIMACY BOOSTERS Studies show that postmenopausal women often have better, more-frequent sex and fewer sexual symptoms when they have a new lover. This underlines the fact that novelty, excitement and emotional closeness can increase sexual intimacy. If you've been in a relationship for a while, you may have to fight to get those feelings back, rather than just looking for a lubricant. Focus on rekindling some magic with your partner:

Make your partner a priority Take time to enjoy each other. Spend some time nurturing your relationship. Go for a long walk or bike ride together. Make a date night at your favorite restaurant. Solve the Saturday crossword puzzle together. For women, all of these things are good foreplay.

If this doesn't fit the definition of foreplay you're used to, consider this analogy: When it comes to sex, most men are like frying pans, ready to sizzle at any time. Most women, on the other hand, are like crockpots. They need to simmer throughout the day spurred on by a morning kiss, a funny midday text exchange, an evening walk or a shared dinner. All of these things can help you feel more connected to your partner, which can lead to better sexual intimacy.

Make sex a priority Try to have sex more often. Plan an overnight trip, so you have time to rediscover one another without the distractions of home and work. Or set aside time at home when both of you like to have sex. That might mean changing your schedule so that you can have sex in the morning when you're both well-rested.

In general, your vagina will lose elasticity if you don't use it. "Not now" may turn into "not ever." In contrast, regular sexual activity can increase blood flow to your vagina and help keep tissues healthy. Just remember that you shouldn't tolerate painful sex. If you have pain during intercourse, prioritize other ways to be sexual while you treat the source of your pain.

Communicate your needs Take time to understand the physical and emotional changes that you and your partner are facing and how they impact your sexual needs. You should be able to talk about sex just like you talk about finances or housework. However, both men and women often have difficulty expressing their sexual preferences out loud. If you're struggling to talk about your desires and needs, start by talking about what you don't want. Which positions no longer feel good? What time of day would you prefer not to have sex? What don't you like about your body? This is often an easier way to start talking about sex, and the conversation can broaden from there.

Good sexual communication is the process of realizing that you can share your desires with your partner without judgment. Talking with your partner can strengthen your sexual relationship and your overall connection. Good communication is also associated with higher sexual satisfaction. If you need help, consider scheduling an appointment with a counselor or sex therapist.

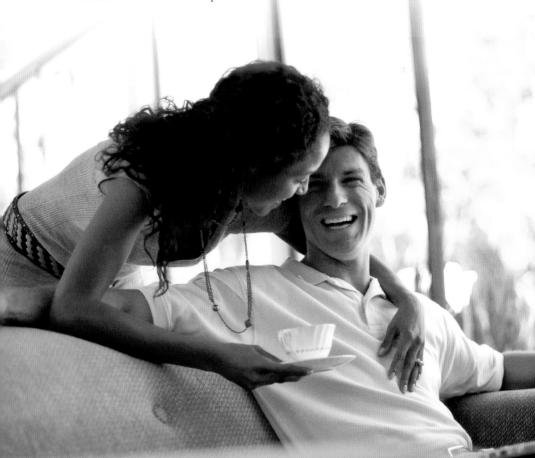

Sensate focus exercises

The goal of sensate focus is not to experience erotic feelings or even feelings of pleasure. Rather, it's meant to help you learn about your own bodily responses and feelings. It can also help you tune into your body by focusing on sensations and bringing attention back to your body when your mind is active or distracted.

In addition, sensate focus can help you accept both giving and receiving. It shows that touching can be just as intimate as intercourse — sometimes even more so — aiding couples to feel close and connected. Ultimately, a couple may experience that erotic feelings eventually arise from touch without pressure.

Instructions for sensate focus

1. Arrange for one hour of complete privacy when you are not exhausted. Relax together first, then have one person touch the other for five to 15 minutes, then switch.

2. Set the mood for relaxation by sitting on the couch together, perhaps sharing a meal. Mood music and low lighting are OK.

3. The temperature should be arranged for comfort.

4. Alcohol or recreational drug use is not suggested.

5. Clothing should be off as much as possible, electronics off and pets elsewhere.

6. Using hands and fingers only, focus your attention on the sensations of temperature, texture and pressure as you touch your partner for your interest, not for his or her pleasure.

7. Do this without words, kissing or full body contact.

Pay particular attention to:

Temperature. Where is your partner warmer or cooler? Does that change?

Texture. Of hair, of skin. Where are they smoother and rougher? What are the textures?

Pressure. How does it feel to you when you use a firmer or lighter touch?

Tips for the *giver*

1. Position your body in order to comfortably touch your partner.

2. Initiate by saying "I'd like to touch now." The receiver can decline, but he or she is then to set another time.

3. Be concerned with your own feelings and sensations rather than those of your partner. Trust that your partner will protect you from doing anything uncomfortable by communicating that to you — nonverbally if possible.

4. Bring any wandering thoughts back to temperature, texture and pressure. If your mind continues to wander, decide how to manage it or stop.

5. Touch long enough to get over any initial feelings of discomfort, but not so long as to get tired or bored (three to five minutes at a minimum).

Tips for the *receiver*

1. Get as relaxed as possible. Begin in any position that's comfortable, and move as you wish.

2. Focus on your feelings coming in, and don't be concerned with what your partner is experiencing. Bring yourself back from distractions and protect your partner by acknowledging — nonverbally if possible — if something is psychologically or physically uncomfortable.

After the exchange of touch, spend time as a couple talking about the experience and any positive and negative feelings that accompanied it. Sensate focus exercises should be made a priority one or two times a week.

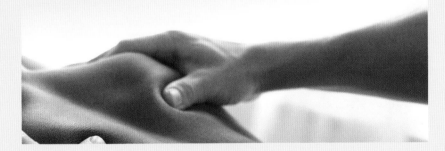

Take it slow If your partner wants to have sex as soon as he gets an erection, you are likely being deprived of the extended foreplay that you need to feel aroused and satisfied. Try slowing things way down.

If you're not sure how, try sensate focus exercises. These exercises involve a series of progressive touching activities designed to help build intimacy. Sensate focus exercises generally follow four phases. In the first two phases, you and your partner focus on touching and caressing each other and exploring the sensations and emotions that you feel. In the third phase, you may add in nonpenetrative sexual activities, followed by penetrative sexual activities in the fourth phase. Sensate focus exercises are a good way for you and your partner to schedule quality, intimate time together. They purposely take away the pressure of penetrative sex and orgasm and help you become comfortable with physical intimacy. See pages 118-119 for instructions.

Venture beyond your usual Try having sex in new positions or different rooms in your house — or outside your house (perhaps a hotel, your backyard or the back of your car). Buy some new lingerie. Plan an erotic surprise, such as a candlelit bath for two or a racy movie. Rekindle your sense of daring and excitement.

Broaden your definition of sex Many couples define sex as penile-vaginal penetration. That's a very narrow definition. There are many other ways to be sexual and sensual. If you have vaginal pain and your partner has erectile problems, you're going to have to rethink what "sex" means for your relationship. If you're not having problems with penetration, you may still find it enjoyable to broaden your horizons as you age.

Need some ideas? The short list might include giving or getting a hickey, tickling, massage, dry humping, masturbating in front of your partner, mutual masturbation, oral sex, manual sex (with hands or fingers), or allowing your partner to ejaculate on your stomach. Biting, spanking, blindfolds, toys and objects that restrict movement also can be part of a satisfying nonpenetrative sexual encounter. Not "going all the way" doesn't have to be G-rated. In fact, taking penetration off the table can force you to be more adventurous and creative, which can also enhance arousal.

Share the work of having good sex If you're struggling with menopausal symptoms, you may be exhausted at the "chore" of figuring out how to rehab your sex life. Shoulder the load with your partner. Split the duties of buying lubricants or a vibrator or scheduling an appointment with a sex therapist. It takes two to tango.

LUBRICANTS, MOISTURIZERS AND VIBRATORS Many couples find that lubricants are a must for midlife sex. If you haven't needed a lubricant before, don't be timid about trying it now. Relying on a bottle for adequate lubrication is not a failure on your part — or your partner's.

Vaginal lubricants reduce the friction associated with thin, dry genital tissue. They're an effective way to provide temporary relief from vaginal dryness and pain before and during sex.

Steer clear of oil-based lubricants (such as petroleum jelly or baby oil); they can cause vaginal irritation and are not compatible with latex condoms. Instead, choose a water- or silicone-based lubricant. The silicone version lasts longer and is generally slicker, which may be good if you have significant vaginal dryness. Silicone lubricants may also be better for water play and for anal sex. However, if you use a sex toy made of silicone, the silicone lubricant will degrade the silicone toy. In addition, the long-lasting extra-slipperiness of a silicone-based lubricant may be enjoyable for you, but this can negatively affect your partner's erection, especially if he has trouble with erectile dysfunction. In these cases, water-based lubricants may be better.

Many women are hesitant to use lubricants, because they believe pausing to worry about gel can kill the moment. However, there are many ways to make adequate lubrication part of your sexual activity, rather than a disruption to the main event. For best results, you'll want lubricant in your vagina, on your vulva and on your partner's penis right before sex. Experiment with applying lubricant on one another as part of your foreplay. Your partner may also enjoy watching you apply lubricant.

If you have vaginal dryness, GSM, arousal difficulties or pain during sex, you may also need a vaginal moisturizer. You apply this product several times a week to moisturize vaginal tissues over time. This can provide longer term relief from vaginal dryness. However, you'll still need a vaginal lubricant right before sex.

Vibrators are another thing to stash in your nightstand drawer, next to the lubricant. As your vagina and clitoris become less sensitive over time, you may need more stimulation to achieve arousal and orgasm. This is where a vibrator comes in handy.

Look for a silicone, battery-powered version that can be used for internal and external stimulation. Try it out on your own before you bring it into bed with your partner. There is no wrong way to use a vibrator. You can use it all over your vulva, thighs, clitoris and other erogenous zones. Experiment with different intensities and areas of your body to see what feels good to you. If you have a waterproof vibrator, the bathtub can be a relaxing, private space to practice. Once you're comfortable, introduce the vibrator into your relationship and show your partner what you like. The more you practice on your own and teach your partner, the easier it will be for you to reach orgasm. Your vibrator can also be used to stimulate your partner.

If vibrators seem risqué to you or you're concerned that they don't align with your values, give it some thought. What are your sexual values? Do you value monogamy? Do you value mutual sexual pleasure? What else? List your values and think about whether a vibrator fits in or not. Many women decide that using a vibrator with a committed partner in a consensual, enjoyable way is actually in line with their sexual values.

Medications

If you can't get sufficient relief from the measures above, you may benefit from a prescription medication. Many medications for sexual symptoms are also remedies for other symptoms of menopause and are discussed in greater detail in Part Three of this book. But here's a brief overview.

ESTROGEN Since declining estrogen is at the heart of vaginal dryness related to menopause, it's no surprise that estrogen can help restore vaginal moisture and reduce pain with sex. It's unclear if estrogen can help boost libido and sex drive.

Estrogen can be delivered throughout your whole body (systemic) by pill, patch, spray or gel. However, there are some risks associated with this form. As a result, systemic estrogen is typically reserved for women who need it to treat other menopause symptoms, such as hot flashes and night sweats.

If vaginal dryness is your only symptom, a smaller doss of estrogen concentrated right where you need it — in the form of a vaginal cream or a slow-releasing suppository or ring that you place in your vagina — is a better option. These forms can restore blood flow to the vagina and improve the suppleness and stretchiness of vaginal tissues in postmenopausal women. Low-dose vaginal estrogen can also reverse thinning and dryness and provide longer term relief than do vaginal lubricants or moisturizers. All of these benefits come without the risks associated with systemic estrogen. You'll need a prescription for any form of vaginal estrogen.

A vaginal cream is applied in the vagina in small amounts two to three times a week. Use it at least 12 hours before sex with your partner. You may still need to use a vaginal lubricant right before sex.

A vaginal tablet is placed into your vagina twice a week using an applicator or your finger. The tablet dissolves inside your vagina.

A low-dose vaginal ring is inserted into your vagina and worn for three months before being removed and replaced. (*Note:* There is also a ring that delivers a systemic dose of estrogen. Don't confuse a low-dose vaginal ring with a systemic estrogen ring.)

Another option is the drug ospemifene (Osphena). This medication is approved to treat moderate to severe pain during sex caused by vaginal dryness or vulvodynia. Ospemifene acts like estrogen on the vaginal lining in some ways, but the risks are not quite the same. However, hot flashes may be a side effect.

TESTOSTERONE Traditionally, testosterone has been referred to as a male sex hormone. But testosterone is essential for physical and mental well-being in women as well. In particular, testosterone has been to shown to improve sexual interest, desire and orgasm in some postmenopausal women.

Prescription testosterone skin patches and gels developed for men contain doses that are inappropriately high for women. However, topical testosterone is sometimes prescribed for women in certain circumstances. These include women with diagnosed low sexual desire with no underly-

When your partner has erectile dysfunction

Erectile dysfunction (impotence) is the inability to get and keep an erection firm enough for sex. It's common in older men.

If you're fortunate enough not to have sexual problems of your own, your partner's erectile dysfunction can still be a problem, leaving you both frustrated and dissatisfied.

If you're struggling with vaginal dryness or sexual pain, your problems may actually be contributing to your partner's sexual dysfunction. Similarly, his problems may be adding to your problems with arousal or orgasm. It can be a cycle. Treating your partner's erectile problems can be a critical step in improving your sexual satisfaction.

Ironically, the cure can bring about a new set of issues. If you haven't had intercourse for a while due to erectile dysfunction, your vagina may have lost some of its elasticity and lubrication. You may not be ready for the sudden restoration of your partner's erections.

It's a good thing that erectile dysfunction medications work so well for so many men. But you and your partner may need to ease back into the saddle and learn how to be sexually active again in a way that is pleasurable for both of you.

Straight talk about safe sex

If you're having sex of any kind with new sexual partners or with a partner who has other partners, protection is a priority.

In fact, if you've been through menopause and you're not using some form of estrogen, your vaginal tissue may be more vulnerable to a sexually transmitted infection (STI) than it was before menopause. That's because the vaginal walls can be thinner and more delicate after menopause, leaving them prone to small tears and cuts that can act as pathways for infection.

If you haven't thought about contraception for a while, here's a refresher on how to have safer sex:

Choose sex partners carefully. Ideally, you should both get tested for STIs before having sex. If that's not going to happen, then it's critical to discuss sexual history with your partner. Thinking or hoping your partner doesn't have an STI is no protection — don't let embarrassment compromise your health.

Insist that male partners always use a new latex condom for each sex act. Do this until you're sure that your partner is disease-free and your relationship has developed into a long-term, mutually monogamous thing. Condoms aren't foolproof, but they're highly effective for reducing transmission of some STIs when used correctly.

Use dental dams. A dental dam is a thin square of latex rubber that you place over your vagina to enjoy oral sex without exchange of bodily fluids. It should be used for oral sex with female partners.

Have an annual physical examination, and get screened for STIs. Sexual infections often have no signs or symptoms until serious complications develop, so regular testing is the best way to detect a problem. Also talk to your doctor about other ways to protect yourself from STIs. You may need a Pap test and HPV testing or a hepatitis B vaccine, if yours isn't up to date.

Limit your cocktails. When you're under the influence of too much alcohol, you're more likely to take sexual risks. Think about all of the advice that you've given your daughters or other young women about sex over the years. Then be sure to heed it in the heat of the moment.

ing cause and women who have low testosterone levels due to certain health conditions or surgical menopause.

There are still concerns about the long-term safety and effectiveness of testosterone in women. In addition, testosterone may cause side effects, such as acne and facial hair. It's important to weigh the benefits and risks.

FLIBANSERIN The medication flibanserin (Addyi) — approved by the FDA in 2015 — has been touted as the female Viagra. However this drug doesn't work like Viagra — it doesn't affect blood flow. But it's approved to treat a small select group of premenopausal women who have been diagnosed with low sexual desire in whom the switch is just turned off for no apparent reason. This drug is not recommended for women who drink alcohol, take certain medications that are metabolized by the liver or have liver impairment.

Be patient with yourself

Ever since Viagra burst onto the marketplace nearly two decades ago and revolutionized sex for older men, women have been clamoring for their own little pink pill. However, no truly comparable drug exists.

How can this gender gap exist? The simple answer is that the female sexual response is complicated. As you learned earlier in this chapter, sexual desire for women depends not just on blood flow and biological issues but also on psychological issues, relationship issues and life issues. It's difficult to fix the whole package with one little pill. In addition, the female sexual response is far more subjective and less measurable than the quality of a penile erection, so it's tough to prove that any new medication actually produces a meaningful sexual effect that is worth any potential side effects.

In the meantime, be patient with yourself. If the entire pharmaceutical industry hasn't found a cure-all for women's sexual dysfunction, with millions of dollars on the line, you can't possibly be expected to remedy your own problems overnight.

Take it slow. Take time to identify your symptoms and try out various self-care measures and other treatments that can help. You can have satisfying sex long after menopause, especially if you're willing to adjust your ideas about sex and try new things. It may not be exactly as it was in your younger years, but it can be equally pleasurable and even mind-blowing.

CHAPTER EIGHT

Incontinence and other pelvic problems

The hormone estrogen has wide-ranging effects. During perimenopause and menopause, when estrogen production begins to decline, a number of changes can take place in a woman's body. In addition to the conditions discussed in previous chapters — such as hot flashes, difficulty sleeping and changes in sexual desire — menopause may lead to changes in your urinary system, resulting in bladder control problems and greater susceptibility to urinary tract infections. If you haven't been bothered by bladder problems before, this can be frustrating. Fortunately, there are many options for treating and managing urinary conditions. Bladder-related troubles shouldn't in any way slow you down or interfere with your daily life.

Just the opposite, other conditions that plague some women during their reproductive years, such as uterine fibroids and heavy menstrual bleeding, typically improve during perimenopause and menopause. If you continue to experience vaginal bleeding or pelvic pressure or pain during menopause, it's important to see your health care provider to determine the cause of your symptoms.

An anatomy lesson

To better understand urinary incontinence and other pelvic conditions, it helps to have some basic knowledge of key organs and structures.

URINARY TRACT Your urinary system has two main parts — upper and lower. The upper urinary tract consists of two kidneys, each attached to a long, muscular tube called a ureter. The kidneys are your body's primary filtration system, removing excess fluid and waste from your bloodstream to make urine. The ureters carry the urine to the bladder, delivering it in small, steady amounts.

Your lower urinary tract consists of the bladder, a slender drainage tube at the bladder's base called the urethra, and two ringlike bands of muscles at the junction of the bladder and the urethra known as the internal and external urethral sphincters. Nerves carry signals from your bladder to your brain to let you know when your bladder is full. Your brain responds back to your bladder when it's time to urinate.

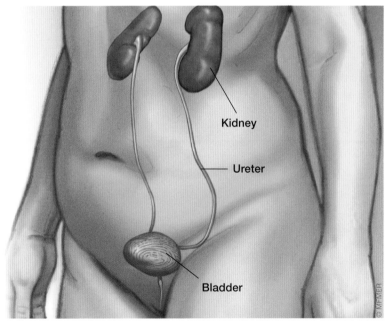

The upper urinary tract consists of two kidneys, each attached to a long, muscular tube called a ureter. Your lower urinary tract consists of the bladder and two ringlike bands of muscles known as the urethral sphincters.

When you urinate, your bladder muscle contracts, pushing urine out of the bladder and through the urethra. The urethral sphincters help control the release of urine. The internal sphincter, composed of muscles that you can't control, keeps your urethra closed while your bladder is filling. The external sphincter, operated by muscles that you can control, helps you keep your urethra closed until you can get to a bathroom. At that time, both sphincters relax, allowing urine to flow out of the bladder and into the urethra.

PELVIC FLOOR MUSCLES Playing a supporting role in the storage and release of urine are the pelvic floor muscles. This hammock-like network of muscles extends from your pubic bone in the front of your pelvis to your tailbone at the base of your spine. The muscles also extend sideways and attach to the inside of your pelvic bones.

Strong pelvic floor muscles are very important for normal bladder function. When you urinate, the pelvic floor muscles relax, allowing urine to pass out of your body easily. When you're not urinating, the pelvic floor muscles lightly contract, holding urine in. These muscles have a number of other functions. They help support your abdominal organs and your back, they

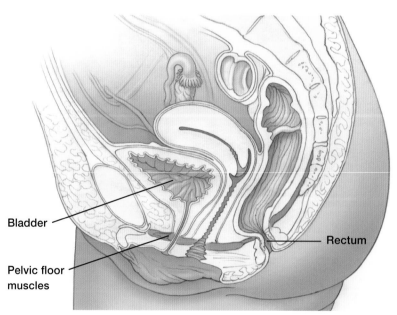

Bladder

Rectum

Pelvic floor muscles

© MFMER

The pelvic floor muscles are a hammock-like network of muscles that extends from your pubic bone in the front of your pelvis to your tailbone at the base of your spine.

contract and relax in order to maintain normal bowel function, and they help make sexual intercourse satisfying and pleasurable. Because these muscles are under voluntary control, they can be strengthened with exercise.

FEMALE REPRODUCTIVE SYSTEM The female reproductive system is composed of those organs associated with childbearing. It's largely located behind the bladder and just above the pelvic floor. This system consists of two ovaries, two fallopian tubes, the uterus and the external genitals.

The ovaries produce the hormones estrogen, progesterone and testosterone and house the female eggs (ova). Each month during ovulation, one of the ovaries releases an egg into the adjacent fallopian tube. The egg travels down the tube and into the uterus.

The uterus is a pear-shaped organ with thick walls, primarily composed of powerful muscles. When a fertilized egg reaches the uterus, it implants itself within the uterine wall and begins to develop into a baby. If the egg isn't fertilized, it degenerates and the lining of the uterus is shed during menstruation. The narrow neck of the uterus, which opens (dilates) to allow the passage of a baby, is called the cervix.

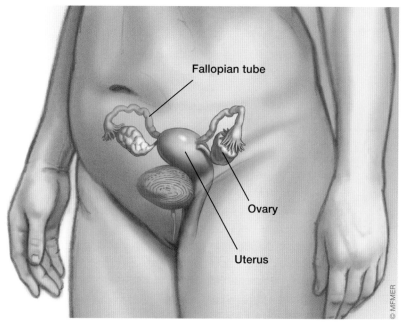

The female reproductive system consists of two ovaries, two fallopian tubes, the uterus and the external genitals.

The external genitals — the mons pubis, labia majora and labia minora, clitoris, and vaginal opening (vestibule) — are called the vulva. These structures are composed mainly of fatty tissue. They also contain glands that secrete substances to lubricate the vaginal opening.

Urinary tract infections

Urinary tract infections (UTIs) are a well-known problem for millions of women. You may have first experienced a UTI when you became sexually active. Perhaps you didn't experience a UTI for several years after learning a few basic steps to help prevent such infections. Now, as you enter menopause, you're experiencing UTIs again, and you may be wondering why.

During menopause and in the years that follow, some women experience an increase in frequency of UTIs. This is because changes in hormone levels during menopause can cause urethral tissues to become more vulnerable to infection. You're also more likely to experience UTIs after menopause if you battled recurrent UTIs in your younger years or if you have a health condition that increases your susceptibility to infection, such as diabetes.

Infection limited to your urethra and bladder can be painful and annoying. However, serious consequences can occur if the infection spreads to your kidneys. So, if you experience signs and symptoms of a UTI — a strong and frequent urge to urinate, a burning sensation when you urinate, urine that appears cloudy or has a strong odor — don't ignore them.

GETTING TREATMENT Antibiotics are typically used to treat UTIs. The type of drug prescribed and how long you need to take it will depend on the type of bacteria found in your urine and your overall health. Usually, symptoms clear within a couple of days. Make sure to take the entire course of antibiotics prescribed by your health care provider to ensure that the infection is completely gone.

If UTIs become a frequent problem, your health care provider may recommend a longer course of antibiotic treatment. If your infections are related to sexual activity, he or she may recommend that after sexual intercourse you take a single dose of an antibiotic.

Another option to help minimize UTIs is vaginal estrogen therapy. Vaginal estrogen helps restore the health of urinary tract tissues, making them less vulnerable to infection. It's also thought to encourage the production of infection-fighting substances in the bladder. Vaginal estrogen is available in the form of a cream, a small tablet inserted into the vagina or a ring.

Straight talk about cranberry juice

There's some indication, though it hasn't been proved, that cranberry juice may have infection-fighting properties, and drinking it daily may help prevent UTIs. Studies have shown the greatest effect in women who have frequent UTIs. It's not clear how much cranberry juice you'd need to drink or how often you'd need to drink it to have an effect. If you like cranberry juice and you feel it helps prevent UTIs, there's little harm in continuing to drink it, but watch the calories. For most people, drinking cranberry juice is safe, but some people report an upset stomach or diarrhea.

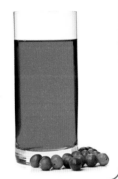

With vaginal therapy, a small amount of estrogen is absorbed into the bloodstream, but much less than with oral (systemic) estrogen therapy. The absorption generally happens in the first few weeks of treatment when the tissues are very thin and dry. After vaginal tissue become more plump and full, absorption of estrogen in the bloodstream is thought to be minimal. As a result, there's a much lower risk of potential side effects.

Understanding incontinence

Another urinary problem that becomes more common around the time of menopause is incontinence, the leakage of urine as a result of decreased bladder control. If you've dealt with this problem, you know that it can be frustrating and embarrassing. But don't let embarrassment get the better of you. Incontinence can be treated, so it's important to discuss your situation with your health care provider.

Urinary incontinence is common. About half of women who are middle-aged and older experience some degree of incontinence at some point in their lives. There are a number of reasons women are bothered by incontinence. First off, a woman's urethra is much shorter than a man's. That means urine has a shorter distance to travel to cause leakage.

Types of incontinence

Not all incontinence is the same. Bladder leakage can occur for different reasons. The most common types of incontinence include:

▶ **Stress incontinence.** Urine leaks when you exert pressure on the bladder by coughing, laughing, exercising or lifting something heavy.

▶ **Urge incontinence.** You have a sudden, intense urge to urinate followed by an involuntary loss of urine. You may need to urinate often, including throughout the night. These symptoms are often referred to as an overactive bladder.

▶ **Overflow incontinence.** You experience frequent or constant dribbling of urine due to a bladder that doesn't empty completely.

▶ **Mixed incontinence.** You have more than one type of incontinence.

Pregnancy and childbirth They can weaken or damage the pelvic floor muscles, which support the uterus, bladder and bowel. Pregnancy and childbirth can also weaken the urethral sphincters. In addition, childbirth can damage nerves in the pelvis, affecting the overall function of the pelvic floor muscles. Oftentimes, the nerve damage doesn't become noticeable until later in life when women begin to lose muscle mass. The change in muscle mass tips the scale enough to cause leakage of urine.

Family history Women whose mothers or older sisters are incontinent are more likely to develop urinary incontinence.

Menopause Some studies suggest a direct link between decreased production of estrogen and the development of incontinence. The decline in estrogen associated with menopause is thought to affect the organs and tissues of the lower urinary tract. The linings of the bladder and urethra become less elastic and are less able to stay closed. Because of these changes, the urethral sphincters (internal and external) may not be able to hold urine as easily as they once did, resulting in urine leakage. But not all studies agree with this theory. Instead, they point to natural aging as the main reason women become incontinent.

Aging Urinary incontinence isn't a normal part of aging — that is, it doesn't naturally occur in all individuals — but it is more common with age.

As you get older, the muscles in your bladder and urethra can lose some of their strength. Because of this, your bladder may not be able to hold as much urine as it once did, meaning you have to urinate more often. And if you don't heed the bathroom call promptly enough, leakage can occur.

In addition, with age your pelvic floor muscles may weaken, making it more difficult to hold in urine. Some research also suggests that your bladder muscle can become overactive as you age. An overactive bladder muscle creates the urge to urinate, even when your bladder isn't full.

Weight gain In general, the more you weigh, the more likely you are to experience urinary incontinence. Being significantly overweight puts increased pressure on your bladder and surrounding muscles, structures and nerves, weakening them and allowing urine to leak, especially when you cough or sneeze. This type of incontinence is known as stress incontinence.

Weight gain is a common problem among women going through perimenopause and menopause. If your weight has increased and you're finding yourself dealing with more problems related to bladder control, there may be a link between the two.

What's important to know is that incontinence can occur for several reasons, and among many women it's likely a combination of factors that leads to its development.

Relief from bladder problems

No matter how bothersome your symptoms are — whether your incontinence is more of an annoyance or it's severe enough that you're afraid to leave the house without a change of clothing — there are steps you can take to manage or treat the problem. Bladder leakage is not something you need to live with, and it shouldn't keep you from leading an active life.

There are a variety of treatments for incontinence. The one that's best for you depends on the type you have and how much it affects your daily life. Most health care providers begin with conservative treatments that are noninvasive or minimally invasive and that have few side effects. If this approach doesn't work, you and your provider may want to consider additional treatment options.

LIFESTYLE CHANGES It's possible that changes in your daily routine may be the only treatment needed to manage your incontinence. Many times, some fairly easy modifications can improve symptoms.

The types and amount of fluid you drink each day, as well as the types of food you eat, can influence your bladder habits. Too much or too little fluid can lead to or worsen incontinence. Certain foods also can irritate the bladder and increase urinary frequency, urgency and leakage.

Pay attention to fluids Drinking too much fluid can make you urinate more often. Excess fluid also can overwhelm your bladder and create a strong sense of urgency — that feeling of needing to go, now! In general, aim for 40 to 60 ounces of fluid daily (approximately five to seven 8-ounce glasses) spread throughout the day. If you get up several times at night to urinate, try drinking most of your fluids in the morning and afternoon.

Surprisingly, drinking too little fluid can cause problems too. Too little fluid can cause your urine to become overly concentrated with your body's waste products. Concentrated urine can irritate your bladder, increasing the urge and frequency with which you need to go urinate. It may also put you at risk of a urinary tract infection.

Avoid irritating foods and beverages Certain foods and beverages can irritate your bladder. Caffeine and alcohol both act as diuretics, which means they increase urine production. This can lead to problems with needing to go to the bathroom often and quickly.

Consuming too many acidic fruits and fruit juices — orange, grapefruit, lemon, lime — also may irritate your bladder. So may spicy foods, tomato-based products, foods and beverages that contain artificial sweeteners, and carbonated drinks. A few people are bothered by milk and milk products. Why these foods can cause irritation in some people isn't well-understood.

If any of these items are a regular part of your diet, try eliminating them for a week or two and see if your symptoms improve. Cut out only one food or beverage at a time so that you can tell which one might be causing the problem.

Check your medications Some medications, including high blood pressure drugs and heart medications, contribute to incontinence in a variety of ways. They may relax the bladder muscle or the urethral sphincters, cause overproduction of urine, or trigger a chronic cough that can worsen stress incontinence. If you're taking a medication that you think may be contributing to your bladder problems, discuss this with your health care provider.

Lose weight As mentioned earlier, being overweight can increase the pressure on your abdomen and the structures in your pelvis, including your bladder. Losing weight has been shown to improve symptoms of

Make sure it's the right pad

Protective pads can help you stay dry and remain active while you take steps to manage and improve your bladder control problems. Most absorbent pads are no more bulky than normal underwear, and you can wear them easily under everyday clothing.

Make certain you purchase products specifically for urine leakage. Don't use menstrual pads because they don't absorb the urine and keep it away from your skin as well as pads designed for bladder control problems. Also avoid pads that contain dyes or perfumes, which can be irritating to your skin.

Absorbent products for urinary incontinence include liners, pads, disposable underwear and reusable underwear. In addition to pulling the moisture away from your skin, these products help control odor. Look for products with a natural odor-absorbing compound, such as baking soda.

incontinence, especially in women with stress incontinence. In one study in which overweight women with stress incontinence took part in a weight-loss program, the women experienced more than a 70 percent reduction in episodes of urine leakage as their weight decreased.

BEHAVIORAL MODIFICATION In addition to conservative measures, there are a few other strategies that can help relieve bladder control problems. Don't be surprised if your health care provider suggests any of the following techniques.

Bladder training Bladder training is intended to improve symptoms related to needing to go to the bathroom frequently. Its purpose is to delay urination when you get the urge to go. You may start by trying to hold off for 10 minutes every time you feel an urge to urinate. The goal is to lengthen the time between trips to the toilet until you're urinating only every two to four hours.

Double voiding Double voiding is used among women who feel they aren't able to empty their bladders completely when urinating. The process involves urinating, then waiting a few minutes and trying again.

Scheduled toilet trips This technique can help with all forms of incontinence. Instead of waiting for the feeling that you need to go to the bathroom, make it a habit to urinate every two to four hours.

PELVIC FLOOR MUSCLE EXERCISES A big part of relieving incontinence, especially stress incontinence that becomes more common with menopause, is to develop strong and well-coordinated pelvic floor muscles. The pelvic floor muscles help control the release of urine, and like other muscles they can weaken over time as a result of childbirth, surgery and aging. By tightening the muscles, you can improve bladder control and reduce urine leakage. When done properly, pelvic floor muscle exercises, also known as Kegels, can be as effective as medications in improving symptoms, if not more so.

How to do them The first step is to know which muscles to tighten. To determine this, imagine that you're urinating and you need to stop the urine flow. Squeeze and lift your vaginal area without tightening your buttocks or belly. You should sense a pulling in or closing in of your genital area when you squeeze. These are the muscles you want to tighten. One way to determine if you're using the right muscles is to place a finger inside your vagina and then squeeze so that you feel the muscles tightening around your finger.

There are different types of strengthening exercises for your pelvic floor muscles. Some promote muscle endurance, while others are designed for a rapid response.

▶ **Holding (endurance) exercises.** Once you know which muscles are involved, practice tightening (contracting) them every day. Slowly, tighten, lift and draw in your pelvic floor muscles and hold them for a count of 10. Relax, then repeat. At first, you may not be able to tighten a full 10 seconds. Start by holding them for one or two seconds, and gradually increase the contraction time over a period of several weeks. Your goal is to be able to do 10 contractions in a row, holding each contraction for 10 seconds at a time and resting for up to 10 seconds between contractions. Do this exercise three times a day, every day if possible, but no less than four days a week.

▶ **Quick flick (coordination) exercises.** With this variation, you contract and release your pelvic floor muscles without holding the contraction. Quickly tighten them, lift them up and let them go. Do this 10 times in a row. You want to do quick flicks after doing endurance exercises. Try to do them three times a day.

▶ **Urge control exercises.** This technique can be used when you feel a sudden, strong urge to urinate. First, stop and stand very still. Sit down

When the muscles are too tight

Some women experience a condition in which the opposite happens. Instead of relaxing and losing their strength, the pelvic floor muscles become too tight. Called nonrelaxing pelvic floor dysfunction, this condition often develops gradually. It may result from an injury to the pelvic floor due to trauma or surgery. Some cases are thought to result from trying to hold back urine or stool instead of allowing passage when the urge is present. Conditions that cause intercourse to be painful (dyspareunia) may lead to involuntary tightening of the muscles.

Symptoms of nonrelaxing pelvic floor dysfunction generally include pain and problems when passing stool or urinating, pain during or after intercourse, and low back pain. Some women experience symptoms early in life, others not until later on. During menopause, changes in the pelvic floor are common.

If you're experiencing these symptoms, your health care provider may recommend that you see a pelvic physical therapist. A therapist can help you learn how to relax and gently stretch your pelvic floor muscles. Devices sometimes used to help stretch the muscles include dilators and deep heating of tissues (diathermy).

if you can. Contract your pelvic floor muscles and hold the contraction for 10 seconds. Take a deep breath and let the air out. Try to think of something other than going to the bathroom. Contract your muscles again if you need to. When you feel the urge has lessened, walk normally to the bathroom. If the urge happens again on the way, stop and repeat the exercise.

When to do them You can do pelvic floor muscle exercises any time and place: while you're standing by the sink washing dishes, while you're in the car traveling to and from work, when you're watching TV or talking on the phone, or when you're in the shower. A simple way to get started is to do your first round of exercises while getting ready in the morning, with another round after lunch, and the last set of repetitions in the evening while relaxing. If you find yourself forgetting to do the exercises, either because you get too busy during the day or you simply don't remember, there are apps for that! You simply download a specific app to your smartphone, and it will remind you when it's time to exercise.

If you're having troubles If you're finding it difficult to identify and contract the right muscles, your health care provider may suggest that you work with a pelvic physical therapist. When you meet with a therapist, he or she will examine your pelvic floor muscles and experiment with various techniques to help you learn how to contract these muscles. The two of you will set up a plan of care individualized to your specific needs. Treatment options may include education, behavioral modification, muscle exercises, and instruction in breathing and relaxation techniques.

Benefits Studies show that if done correctly, pelvic floor muscle exercises can be effective in reducing or preventing urine leakage when you cough, sneeze or laugh. When you feel a sneeze or cough coming on or you know you're going to laugh, contract your pelvic floor muscles to hold in urine. The exercises can also help hold in urine when you have a sudden urge to go to the bathroom.

Most women begin to notice an improvement after a few weeks of practicing pelvic floor muscle exercises regularly. It's the same as going to the gym; it takes time to build muscle! If you have severe leakage, the exercises may be less helpful, and you may need other forms of treatment to improve your symptoms.

MEDICATIONS Sometimes medications are prescribed to help treat urinary incontinence. In general, medications are more effective for reducing symptoms of urge incontinence than stress incontinence. A class of medications known as anticholinergics may be recommended to help calm an overactive bladder. Examples include the drugs oxybutynin (Ditropan XL), tolterodine (Detrol) and solifenacin (Vesicare).

The drug mirabegron (Myrbetriq) also may be used to treat urge incontinence. It relaxes the bladder muscle and can increase the amount of urine your bladder can hold. It may also increase the amount you're able to urinate at one time, helping to empty your bladder more completely.

A low-dose, topical estrogen in the form of a vaginal cream, ring or tablet may be used to help restore the health of tissues in the urethra and vaginal areas. Topical estrogen is generally more effective in reducing symptoms of urge incontinence than of stress incontinence. Estrogen taken orally in pill form (systemic therapy) isn't effective for treating incontinence.

DEVICES AND INJECTIONS Other treatments for incontinence include devices intended to block urine flow and procedures to bulk up urinary tissues and structures.

Urethral insert Before an activity that can trigger incontinence, such as a game of tennis, you insert a small, tampon-like disposable device into your urethra. The insert acts as a plug to prevent leakage. You remove it when the activity is finished.

Pessary This is a stiff ring that you insert into your vagina and wear all day. The device helps hold up your bladder, which lies in front of the vagina, to prevent urine leakage. You may benefit from a pessary if you have incontinence due to a prolapsed bladder or uterus, a condition in which the structures drop out of their normal positions and protrude into the vagina.

Bulking agents A synthetic material is injected into tissue surrounding the urethra. The bulking material helps keep the urethra closed and reduces urine leakage. This procedure is less effective than more-invasive treatments such as surgery, and it usually needs to be repeated regularly.

OnabotulinumtoxinA (Botox) Injections of Botox into the bladder muscle may benefit people who have an overactive bladder. Botox causes the bladder to relax, increasing its storage capacity and reducing episodes of incontinence. It's generally prescribed only if other first line medications haven't been successful.

SURGERY If other treatments aren't working, surgery may be able to treat the underlying cause of your incontinence. There are several surgical procedures that may be considered, depending on your circumstances and the severity of your symptoms. Surgery offers high cure rates for stress incontinence. It may also bring relief to some women with urge incontinence.

Uterine fibroids

A condition common to a number of women is that of uterine fibroids. These are noncancerous growths of the uterus that often appear during childbearing years. If you've dealt with uterine fibroids, you should begin to notice relief from your symptoms as you enter menopause. During menopause, when normal menstrual bleeding stops and steroid hormone levels decrease, symptoms of uterine fibroids typically improve and the condition gradually disappears.

If your symptoms persist once you've experienced menopause, see your health care provider. Also be aware that use of oral (systemic) hormone therapy during menopause can cause some women to continue to experience problems associated with uterine fibroids, but the symptoms generally are mild.

Uterine fibroids develop from the smooth, muscular tissue of the uterus (myometrium). A single cell divides repeatedly, eventually creating a firm, rubbery mass that's distinct from nearby tissue. Also called leiomyomas or myomas, uterine fibroids aren't associated with an increased risk of uterine cancer. But they can be bothersome.

Fibroids range in size from seedlings, undetectable by the human eye, to bulky masses that can distort and enlarge the uterus. As many as 3 out of 4 women have uterine fibroids sometime during their lives. Most are unaware of the growths because they often don't cause any symptoms. In women who do experience signs and symptoms, the most common are heavy menstrual bleeding, prolonged menstrual periods, pelvic pressure or pain, frequent urination, and troubles with bladder emptying.

Studies of women with a history of uterine fibroids who take hormone therapy to relieve other symptoms of menopause, such as hot flashes, indicate that the therapy generally causes only small fibroid growth and mild symptoms, if any at all. If you experience vaginal bleeding, don't simply chalk it up to fibroids. Make sure to see your health care provider to have it evaluated.

Vaginal bleeding

Once you've completed menopause — that is, you've gone without a period for more than a year — you shouldn't have any menstrual bleeding. After menopause, even a little spotting isn't considered normal. With any type of postmenopausal bleeding, it's important to make an appointment to see your health care provider.

CAUSES A number of conditions may cause vaginal bleeding after menopause. Most of them aren't serious, but some of them are; that's why it's important to know what's behind the blood loss.

Tissue changes The most common reason for postmenopausal bleeding is thinning and drying of tissues that make up the uterus, vagina and vulva. Another name for this condition is genitourinary syndrome of menopause (GSM). Because the surfaces of the tissues contain little moisture after menopause, they may bleed easily. Bleeding may result from intercourse, irritation of the tissues or an infection. In one study, thinning of the tissues of the vagina and uterine lining (endometrium) was responsible for almost 60 percent of postmenopausal bleeding.

Tissue thinning and drying may begin to bother you during the years leading up to menopause, or it may not become a problem until several years into menopause. Some women are never bothered by it.

Polyps and fibroids Benign growths such as uterine polyps and uterine fibroids are another cause of vaginal bleeding. Uterine polyps are growths on the inner wall of the uterus that extend into the uterine cavity. Overgrowth of cells in the lining of the uterus (endometrium) leads to the formation of uterine polyps, also known as endometrial polyps. Uterine polyps most commonly occur in women who are going through or have completed menopause, although younger women can get them, too. Their exact cause is unknown, but hormonal factors appear to play a role.

As mentioned earlier, uterine fibroids are benign growths that often occur during childbearing years that tend to disappear during menopause. Sometimes, however, the condition may continue into menopause, causing postmenopausal bleeding. The main difference between uterine polyps and uterine fibroids is that fibroids are composed of muscle tissue and polyps are made of endometrial tissue.

Hormone therapy A number of women who take estrogen to relieve symptoms of menopause, such as hot flashes and sleep difficulties, experience some vaginal bleeding while taking hormones. The frequency of bleeding depends on the regimen used. If the bleeding is unscheduled — occurring at times in your cycle when you're not expecting it — or it's heavy, talk to your health care provider. Also make an appointment to see your care provider if you experience other bothersome symptoms, such as bloating or pain. You want to make certain the bleeding isn't related to another cause.

Cancer In approximately 5 to 10 percent of women who experience postmenopausal bleeding, the bleeding is a result of endometrial cancer. If endometrial cancer is detected early, surgery to remove the uterus often cures the cancer. If the cancer is more advanced, other treatments may be necessary. Other types of cancer, such as cervical and vaginal cancer, also can cause vaginal bleeding. These cancers are a less common cause of postmenopausal bleeding than is endometrial cancer.

Endometrial hyperplasia Endometrial hyperplasia refers to abnormal growth (thickening) of the uterine lining. In some cases, the condition can lead to cancer of the uterus. Endometrial hyperplasia usually occurs after menopause, when ovulation stops and production of the hormone progesterone declines. It can also occur during perimenopause when ovulation may not occur regularly. Obesity or use of medications that act like estrogen also may lead to the condition.

Abnormal bleeding is the most common sign of endometrial hyperplasia. If you experience abnormal bleeding resulting from the condition, your health care provider will likely suggest treatment to prevent the condition from becoming cancerous. Options include a progestin medication, which may be administered in the form of a pill, shot or intrauterine device (IUD). Another option is surgery to remove the uterus (hysterectomy).

Infection An infection of the uterus, such as endometritis or cervicitis, occasionally can cause bleeding.

EVALUATION Two tests used to help determine the cause of abnormal uterine bleeding are an endometrial biopsy and a transvaginal ultrasound. In an endometrial biopsy, a small sample of the lining of the uterus (endometrium) is removed and examined under a microscope for abnormal cells. An endometrial biopsy may be performed to find the cause of abnormal bleeding, check for overgrowth of the lining (endometrial hyperplasia) or check for cancer.

With a transvaginal ultrasound, an ultrasound probe is placed inside the vagina to look at your reproductive organs and pelvic area. This test may be done to look for abnormalities causing abnormal bleeding, such as polyps and fibroids, or in cases when an endometrial biopsy isn't preferable or possible.

TREATMENT If tests reveal cancer or an increased risk of cancer, surgery may be performed to remove the cancer or the abnormality that's putting you at increased risk, such as with endometrial hyperplasia.

If the condition isn't serious and you aren't experiencing significant symptoms, you may not need any additional treatment. For thinning and drying of vaginal tissues, your health care provider may recommend a vaginal estrogen cream, tablet or ring. These use a much lower dose of estrogen than do oral (systemic) hormone therapies and thus limit your overall exposure to estrogen and its associated risks. Vaginal estrogen therapies help to reverse vulvar and vaginal tissue changes by restoring the vagina's normal pH balance, thickening surface tissue and increasing lubrication. Use of moisturizers to help maintain tissue moisture and lubricants during sexual intercourse also may help (see Chapter 7).

If the bleeding worsens or changes, make sure to see your health care provider as soon as possible.

Going forward

During menopause, a variety of changes may take place. If these changes are difficult or bothersome, don't simply accept them and live with them. Often, conditions associated with menopause can be managed or possibly even eliminated with a few lifestyles changes or interventional therapies. Don't be afraid to speak up and ask questions. You may find the topic a bit embarrassing, but it's likely a conversation your health care provider has had with many other women in the same situation. There's no reason to be ashamed or embarrassed. Once you've taken this important first step, you'll be well on your way to a more relaxed and enjoyable daily routine.

PART THREE

Taking control of your symptoms

CHAPTER NINE

Weight management

··

You might be surprised to see weight management as the first topic under symptom control. But maintaining a healthy weight through a nutritious diet and regular exercise is a key starting point as you seek to manage your symptoms and optimize your health in midlife.

A healthy weight — one in which you have an appropriate amount of body fat compared to your overall body mass — reduces your risk of diseases and gives you energy to live your life. It may also help you better manage your menopausal symptoms like hot flashes and poor sleep. As you learned in the Quick Start guide and Chapter 3, women at midlife usually have to contend with a number of bodily changes such as weight gain, an expanding waistline, muscle loss, and an increased risk of cardiovascular and other diseases. Weight management is a key strategy to combat these trends.

Think of weight management as a baseline approach — setting a solid foundation for any other treatment options you might try. For example, if you do want to consider hormone therapy to manage your symptoms, you need to be generally healthy and free of certain health conditions such as cardiovascular disease.

Even if you're already at a healthy weight, you may find the changes that come with menopause and age make it harder to maintain your weight. Now is a good time to focus on your well-being and form healthy habits that will last you the rest of your life. This chapter will provide you with the knowledge and tools to get started. Weight management is not easy, but the rewards are well worth it for your health and quality of life.

Your healthy weight

How do you know if you're at a healthy weight? To answer that question, you need to consider more factors than just the number on the scale.

The impacts of excess body weight

Excess body weight has serious health implications that can affect your quality of life and longevity. For women entering menopause, being overweight or obese is associated with more frequent hot flashes. And although obesity is generally associated with a lower risk of osteoporosis, this hasn't been found to reduce the risk of fractures. Obesity is also a risk factor for cardiovascular disease — the leading cause of death in women, and a disease that tends to become more prevalent after menopause. Obesity can increase your risk of insulin resistance, type 2 diabetes, high blood pressure, elevated cholesterol levels, stroke, gallbladder disease, liver disease, sleep apnea, osteoarthritis, certain types of cancer and your overall risk of dying. It may also increase the risk of Alzheimer's disease. Your risk of developing these weight-related health problems increases with age. But beyond these disease risks, being obese can also have a significant impact on your overall well-being and self-esteem.

The good news is that you don't need to achieve a bodybuilder's physique in order to improve your health. A weight loss of even 3 to 5 percent of your body weight can start to result in health benefits — and it may reduce the number of hot flashes you experience.

BODY MASS INDEX You're probably familiar with the body mass index (BMI). It's a measure of your body weight in relation to your height. You can find many calculators online that will tell you your BMI. This index has become the routine way to identify obesity. A BMI of 25 or greater is classified as "overweight" and 30 or greater is classified as "obese." However, your BMI doesn't differentiate between weight due to fat mass versus muscle mass. Also, BMI doesn't provide any information about the distribution of excess body fat — whether it is around the belly or in the lower body, or both. BMI and distribution of excess body fat are both important factors that have significant implications for your health.

What's your BMI?

To determine your body mass index (BMI), find your height in the left column. Follow that row across until you reach the column with the weight nearest yours. Look at the top of the column for your approximate BMI.

	Normal		Overweight				Obese				
BMI	**19**	**24**	**25**	**26**	**27**	**28**	**29**	**30**	**35**	**40**	**45**	**50**
Height						Weight in pounds						
4'10"	91	115	119	124	129	134	138	143	167	191	215	239
4'11"	94	119	124	128	133	138	143	148	173	198	222	247
5'0"	97	123	128	133	138	143	148	153	179	204	230	255
5'1"	100	127	132	137	143	148	153	158	185	211	238	264
5'2"	104	131	136	142	147	153	158	164	191	218	246	273
5'3"	107	135	141	146	152	158	163	169	197	225	254	282
5'4"	110	140	145	151	157	163	169	174	204	232	262	291
5'5"	114	144	150	156	162	168	174	180	210	240	270	300
5'6"	118	148	155	161	167	173	179	186	216	247	278	309
5'7"	121	153	159	166	172	178	185	191	223	255	287	319
5'8"	125	158	164	171	177	184	190	197	230	262	295	328
5'9"	128	162	169	176	182	189	196	203	236	270	304	338
5'10"	132	167	174	181	188	195	202	209	243	278	313	348
5'11"	136	172	179	186	193	200	208	215	250	286	322	358
6'0"	140	177	184	191	199	206	213	221	258	294	331	368
6'1"	144	182	189	197	204	212	219	227	265	302	340	378
6'2"	148	186	194	202	210	218	225	233	272	311	350	389
6'3"	152	192	200	208	216	224	232	240	279	319	359	399

Source: National Institutes of Health, 1998
Asians with a BMI of 23 or higher may have an increased risk of health problems.

Despite these limitations, your BMI still provides useful information in understanding whether you're at a healthy weight.

FAT DISTRIBUTION You may have heard about the increased health risks that come with having an "apple-shaped" body type — where fat is carried around the waist — compared to a "pear-shaped" body type — where fat is stored in the hips and thighs. Belly fat, or visceral fat, is stored deeper in your abdomen, surrounding your organs, and affects your body in more adverse ways than does subcutaneous fat, which is stored under your skin. Excess visceral fat is associated with a greater risk of diseases such as type

2 diabetes, hypertension, high cholesterol and higher rates of death —
even in individuals with a normal BMI. Storing fat in your legs
or hips is generally associated with lower cardiovascular risks, even in
individuals classified as obese by the BMI scale.

Genetics plays a role in your fat distribution, and you also tend to store
more fat around your middle as you age. And as you learned in Chapter 3,
the loss of estrogen at menopause is associated with greater fat accumulation around your middle. Measuring your waist circumference is an easy
way to determine whether you are carrying too much belly fat. Using a
flexible measuring tape, stand and measure around your abdomen just
above your hipbone. Pull the tape measure until it's snug but doesn't press
into your skin, and make sure it's level all the way around. For women, a
waist measurement of 35 inches (89 centimeters) or more indicates an
unhealthy concentration of belly fat. However, there is nothing magic about
that particular number. In general, the greater the waist measurement, the
greater the health risks. And though the health impacts of visceral fat are
serious, the good news is that when you lose weight, abdominal fat tends to
be lost first, and at a higher rate than fat elsewhere in your body. Exercise
also plays an important role in targeting visceral fat — more on that later.

BODY COMPOSITION When determining obesity, the BMI scale isn't able
to take into account your body composition, which refers to the relative
percentages of fat and lean muscle mass in your body. Especially in the
middle ranges of the index, it may misdiagnose some individuals as obese
when they actually have a high amount of lean muscle mass and low body
fat. The BMI scale may also classify some individuals as being at a normal
weight when in reality they have too much body fat and a low muscle mass.

This latter condition, termed *normal weight obesity*, has recently received
significant attention. This is because an individual with normal weight
obesity has the same or greater health risks as does someone who's
considered obese according to the BMI scale. Often, normal weight obesity
is combined with excess abdominal fat. This toxic combination leads to
greater cardiovascular risks and the highest risk of death of any group —
even greater than those individuals classified as obese. Individuals with
normal weight obesity are specifically at a greater risk of soft plaques in the
arteries, which can lead to heart attacks. In particular, women who have
normal BMI but a high body fat percentage may be at risk of early death
due to cardiovascular disease.

If you have a BMI within the normal range but are carrying excess body
fat, you will have low muscle mass. And because people tend to lose

muscle and gain fat as they age, the BMI scale's accuracy tends to worsen as you age. Regardless, it's still the case that looking at your BMI alone may mask a trend toward normal weight obesity and cause you to underestimate your cardiovascular risks. Approximately 30 million Americans may be considered normal weight obese and not know it. Fortunately, as with its role in targeting abdominal fat, exercise is one strategy that can help improve body composition and thus reduce the likelihood of normal weight obesity.

PUTTING IT ALL TOGETHER Your BMI, fat distribution and body composition — as well as information about your diet, activity levels, and your family and personal health history — will help you and your health care provider determine your healthy weight. Together, you can discuss any weight-related goals you might have. These goals may include losing fat, building muscle mass, improving your nutrition or all of the above. And, if you and your health care provider determine weight loss is your goal, discuss strategies to do so in a healthy way.

Understanding your energy balance

Weight gain and loss are dependent upon your energy balance — in other words, calories in versus calories expended. Calories from food provide the fuel you need to power your body's basic processes — such as breathing, circulating blood, digestion and physical activity — as well as regulating hormone levels and growing and repairing cells. The calories you need to maintain your current weight depend on a variety of factors, including your sex, age, body size and composition, and activity level.

Though some individuals are genetically predisposed to being overweight, it's ultimately a result of calorie intake exceeding expenditure. The scales have to tip in the other direction in order for you to lose weight. You need to reduce your calorie consumption or increase the amount of calories you burn or both. The healthiest weight loss — and the type you're most likely to maintain — tends to be slow and steady. People sometimes lose weight faster in the first few weeks of losing weight. However, long-term weight loss of about 1 or 2 pounds a week is considered a reasonable goal for most people.

You may have heard that 3,500 calories is the magic number that equals approximately a pound of body fat — meaning you'd have to cut 500 to 1,000 calories a day in order to achieve 1 to 2 pounds of weight loss a week.

The role of diet and exercise in weight management

So what's more important if you want to lose weight — diet or exercise? The answer is that both are equally important, but for different reasons.

Exercise burns calories and is effective in preventing weight gain, even in individuals with a genetic predisposition to obesity. It also improves your body composition, targets visceral fat and has numerous health benefits. However, it's hard to lose weight through physical activity alone. Research indicates that diet is a more critical component of losing weight, at least in the initial stages, and that exercise has a greater impact on keeping the pounds off over time. A combined approach is likely the most effective way to maintain your healthy weight in the long term.

One reason diet plays such a large role in weight loss is because it's much easier to take in calories than it is to expend them. For example, it may only take you a few minutes to eat a 250-calorie snack of crackers and cheese, but it may take you an hour of brisk walking to burn that same number of calories. You can very quickly cancel out the calories burned in a significant amount of exercise with just minor changes in your diet.

If you had hoped that your intense workout routine meant that you didn't have to monitor your diet — or you thought that extreme calorie restriction meant that you could avoid having to exercise — you'll have to think again. Diet and exercise play essential and complementary roles in achieving and maintaining a healthy weight.

While this may be a helpful rule of thumb to get you started, the reality is a lot more complex — primarily on the expenditure side of the equation.

As you lose weight, your body mass and composition change. Your body responds by undergoing a variety of hormonal changes that may make it more challenging to keep the scale going down. And you also have the hormonal shifts of menopause to contend with. After you've lost weight, you tend to burn fewer calories through basic metabolic processes, and your calorie expenditure through exercise also decreases. What this all means is that the same number of calories that originally gave you a negative energy balance may no longer be enough to keep up your weight loss. You may very likely need to cut down your calorie intake further to sustain weight loss.

This is a common experience — the dreaded weight-loss plateau — and it can be a frustrating time. Knowing ahead of time that it will likely occur may help you prepare for it. When you do reach a plateau, it's a good time to reassess your goals and remind yourself why you've committed to losing weight. In order to kick-start your weight loss, you might need to reduce your calorie intake further and rev up your workout routine. Exercise counteracts the decreased energy expenditure that occurs in response to the reduced calorie intake. Take a look at your eating and exercise habits — research has shown that plateaus often happen earlier than they would naturally because of slip-ups in sticking with your healthy practices. Keep in mind that if you are strength training, increased muscle mass may mask fat loss if you're only looking at the number on the scale.

Weight loss is a journey that's best measured in years, not months. Knowing this in advance can help you set reasonable goals and prepare for the long haul and the inevitable bumps in the road.

Foundations of a healthy diet

Though there's always a new fad diet that promises rapid weight loss, the same old advice holds true as you try to reach your weight-related goals: Build from the right foundation.

A BALANCED APPROACH The foundations of healthy eating haven't changed. Focus on eating a healthy and balanced diet based on vegetables, fruits, whole grains and lean proteins, and limit saturated and trans fats, sodium, and added sugar. This sort of diet can improve your health and help you reach your weight goals. It can also be enjoyable — a key element in achieving long-term success. It's important to adopt healthy dietary habits that you can sustain long term, as opposed to changes that you will not be able to adhere to in your weight-loss journey.

The Mayo Clinic Healthy Weight Pyramid can be a helpful tool as you seek to make healthy food choices. Vegetables and fruits form the base of the pyramid, and — with the exception of dried fruits and fruit juice — there's no upper limit to how many servings you can have of these healthy items. The serving recommendations for other food groups depend on your calorie goals. This is the "intake" side of your energy balance equation. A daily goal of 1,200 calories for women is a reasonable starting point if weight loss is your goal — any lower than that and you may not be getting the nutrients you need. No specific food is off-limits, but it needs to fit within your overall healthy-eating plan and your goal of having your calorie expenditure exceed your intake.

FOCUS ON FIBER If you are eating from the base of the Pyramid, you'll already be consuming foods that are low in energy density — that is, they have few calories for their volume. This means you can eat more of them, consume fewer calories and feel fuller. Water and fiber in food help contribute to low energy density, meaning most fruits and vegetables fall under this category.

Fiber is the component of plant-based foods that isn't absorbed by your body. It supports the health of your digestive tract and can reduce insulin resistance as well as the risk of high blood pressure, type 2 diabetes, stroke and heart disease. There's evidence that diets high in fiber are associated with lower body weight.

Unfortunately, most women don't get enough fiber. Try to get 14 grams of fiber for every 1,000 calories in your diet. For example, at age 55, a moderately active woman needs 1,800 calories to maintain weight, and 25 grams of fiber a day. Fiber is found in fruits, vegetables, whole grains, beans, lentils, nuts and seeds. Eat your fruit and vegetables with their skins on to help increase your fiber intake, and drink plenty of water to help fiber move through your digestive tract.

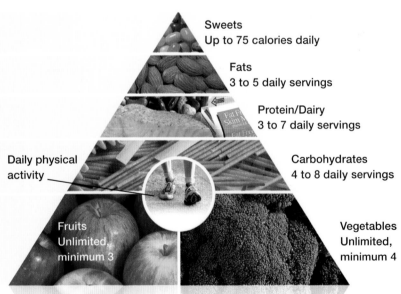

Sweets
Up to 75 calories daily

Fats
3 to 5 daily servings

Protein/Dairy
3 to 7 daily servings

Daily physical activity

Carbohydrates
4 to 8 daily servings

Fruits
Unlimited,
minimum 3

Vegetables
Unlimited,
minimum 4

Mayo Clinic Healthy Weight Pyramid
See your health care provider before you begin any healthy-weight plan.

PORTION DISTORTION A serving of food is a specific measured amount of food. A portion is how much food we put on our plate, and may contain many servings. An important component of weight loss or maintaining a healthy weight is eating moderate portion sizes. "Portion distortion" has become very common, and large portions are so prevalent that it seems normal to consume large amounts of food in a single meal. However, standard portions of food are often much more than your body needs. This distortion is reinforced by the size of our plates, serving utensils and meal packaging.

Take the time to learn about serving sizes and how many you need each day from the different food groups. Visual cues can help you remember and estimate serving sizes in your meals — see below for some examples. And although calculating serving sizes from a dish with more than one ingredient can be more complex, it can be done and will get easier with practice.

Sizing up a serving

It's important to understand how much of a particular food makes up a serving. Many people envision servings to be larger than they are. These visual clues can help you gauge general serving sizes.

Vegetables	Visual cue
1 cup broccoli 2 cups raw, leafy greens	1 baseball 2 baseballs
Fruits	**Visual cue**
½ cup sliced fruit 1 small apple or medium orange	Tennis ball
Starch (carbohydrates)	**Visual cue**
½ cup pasta, rice or dried cereal ½ bagel 1 slice whole-grain bread	Hockey puck
Protein and dairy	**Visual cue**
2½ ounces chicken or fish 1½ ounces beef 2 ounces hard cheese	Deck of cards ½ deck of cards 4 dice
Fats	**Visual cue**
1½ teaspoons peanut butter 1 teaspoon butter or margarine	2 dice 1 die

Be wary of beverages

It's easy to gulp down hundreds of extra calories in a matter of minutes, which is why high-calorie beverages can quickly sabotage your weight-loss goals. Individuals who consume sugary drinks — including fruit juice with added sugar — are at an increased risk of weight gain.

Though you may think diet soda is a better choice if you're trying to lose weight — it says "diet," right? — you might need to think again. One study found that diet soda intake was associated with greater waist circumference and abdominal fat gain — even in the absence of a changing BMI. Though waist circumference tends to increase with age anyway, diet soda consumers had a three times greater gain in waist circumference than nonsoda drinkers. This effect was exacerbated in individuals who were already overweight or obese.

Instead of sugary drinks, focus on getting lots of water. Try adding lemon or cucumber for some flavor without the calories, or try sparkling water if you need a bit of fizz. If high-calorie coffee drinks are your downfall,try a low-fat milk, such as 1 percent or skim, skip the whipped cream and try to find a satisfying, low-calorie alternative most of the time.

And don't forget alcohol, another source of concentrated calories. Alcohol has been associated with more fat being stored around the abdomen. If you drink, do so in moderation — up to one drink a day for women is considered a reasonable amount. However, it is probably not a good idea to have a drink every day if you're concerned about your weight.

Exercise at menopause

The importance of exercise for menopausal women can't be overstated. At a time in life when your disease risk is often creeping up and you have a harder time managing your weight, exercise can be an invaluable tool in your toolbox.

THE POWER OF EXERCISE Exercise can play a unique role in combating two common trends experienced around menopause — loss of muscle mass and an expanding waistline. Exercise builds muscle, improving your body composition and making it less likely you'll fall into the category of normal weight obesity. Greater muscle mass helps your body burn more calories at rest and during exercise. And though weight loss by either diet or exercise seems effective in reducing abdominal fat, exercise seems to play a more important role. Some research shows that strength training can lead to a reduction in abdominal fat — even without a change in overall body weight or BMI. And you don't have to be a fitness addict to see benefits — both moderate- and vigorous-intensity exercise can reduce visceral fat. Continuing to exercise after weight loss can specifically help prevent you from regaining belly fat.

Regardless of your BMI, exercise lowers the risk of death and reduces your risk of many diseases such as osteoporosis and cardiovascular disease — conveying important health benefits even while you may still be working on shedding pounds. Although it's hard to lose weight through physical activity alone, exercise does play an important role in preventing weight gain in the first place, as well as maintaining the weight loss achieved through calorie restriction.

By helping you maintain a healthy weight, exercise may help manage your menopausal symptoms. Though studies are conflicting as to whether exercise helps reduce hot flashes, regular exercise can improve sleep, relieve anxiety and stress, enhance sexual arousal, and improve your overall quality of life. If you aren't used to exercising, it may initially be a trigger for hot flashes because it increases your core body temperature. If your hot flashes are bothersome, you may want to start slowly and pick up the pace as your fitness increases.

HOW MUCH DO YOU NEED? Current U.S. guidelines recommend adults get at least 150 minutes of moderate-intensity aerobic exercise or 75 minutes of vigorous aerobic activity a week for health benefits and to maintain weight. This is equal to 30 minutes of moderate-intensity activity five days out of the week. Even greater health benefits will come from getting 300 minutes of moderate-intensity or 150 minutes of vigorous aerobic activity — and this higher amount is likely needed in order to lose weight and keep it off.

It's also important to include strength training activities at least twice a week. This is especially true for menopausal women who are trying to prevent muscle loss and maintain bone strength. There are many options for muscle strengthening exercises — you can use weight machines, hand-held weights, resistance bands or your own body weight. Consider finding a reputable personal trainer to get started with strength training activities if you aren't familiar with them. Balance and flexibility exercises can round out your exercise routine and help improve your stability and range of motion.

Exercise for multiple benefits

Exercise has a number of benefits in addition to helping you maintain a healthy weight. Exercise can:

▶ Build lean muscle mass, improving strength and increasing your metabolism
▶ Reduce visceral fat
▶ Slow the bone loss that comes with menopause and reduce the risk of falls and osteoporosis
▶ Decrease insulin resistance and reduce your risk of various diseases, such as heart disease, type 2 diabetes, high blood pressure, and breast and colon cancers — and exercise can function as a treatment for many of these same conditions
▶ Stimulate your brain and perhaps even reduce the risk of cognitive decline and Alzheimer's disease
▶ Boost your mood and combat depression
▶ Enhance sexual arousal
▶ Improve sleep and energy levels

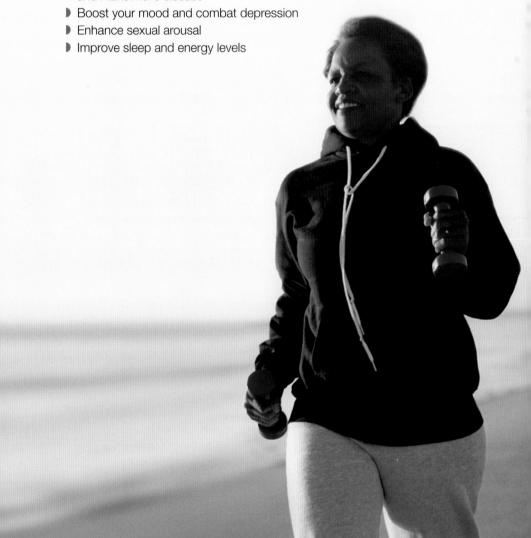

If you haven't exercised in a while, or if you have a health condition that prevents you from meeting these recommendations — talk to your health care provider before starting a new activity. Be as active as your health allows, and remember that something is always better than nothing! And while the recommended amounts might sound daunting, breaking up your activity throughout the week will make it more manageable. Make sure to keep your routine varied — an exercise plan pairing aerobic activity plus strength training tends to be the most effective for reducing body weight, waist circumference, overall fat mass and visceral fat.

Create lasting change

Achieving and maintaining a healthy weight is no quick fix. It requires developing positive lifelong behaviors — and strategies to continually reinforce these behaviors — that will help you succeed in reaching your goals. This is why it's important to keep your motivation for change front and center in your mind. Whatever it is that you value — whether it's being able to live independently and travel long into your golden years or being a healthy role model for your kids and grandkids — this is the fuel for your commitment to lasting change.

Weight-loss success has more to do with sticking to a plan than choosing a specific diet. It will take commitment, planning and time to develop your weight management strategies and systems that will allow you to overcome the barriers and behaviors that led you to gain weight in the first place. However, while it takes time, effort and changes in habits to successfully lose and then maintain weight, the return on investment in your health and quality of life can be tremendous. Here are some tips to help you get started.

SET REALISTIC GOALS

▶ Set realistic goals so that you don't get discouraged, and remember that change takes perseverance and time. Unrealistic goals make it less likely that you'll adhere to your healthy behaviors.

▶ Goals will be most effective if they are aligned with your values. Remember that weight loss is a means to an end. Reflecting on your values and why you committed to losing weight in the first place can help renew your motivation and reinforce healthy behaviors when the going gets tough.

Sitting — The new smoking

Research has linked sitting for long periods of time with a number of health concerns, including obesity and metabolic syndrome — a cluster of conditions that includes increased blood pressure, high blood sugar, excess body fat around the waist and abnormal cholesterol levels. Too much sitting also seems to increase the risk of death from cardiovascular disease and cancer.

Sitting in front of the TV isn't the only concern. Any extended sitting — such as behind a desk at work or behind the wheel — can be harmful. What's more, spending a few hours a week at the gym or otherwise engaging in moderate or vigorous activity doesn't seem to significantly offset the risk.

The solution seems to be less sitting and more moving overall. You might start by simply standing rather than sitting whenever you have the chance or think about ways to walk while you work. For example:

▶ Stand while talking on the phone or eating lunch.

▶ If you work at a desk for long periods of time, try a standing desk — or improvise with a high table or counter.

▶ Walk laps with your colleagues rather than gathering in a conference room for meetings.

▶ Position your work surface above a treadmill — with a computer screen and keyboard on a stand or a specialized treadmill-ready vertical desk — so that you can be in motion throughout the day.

The impact of movement — even leisurely movement — can be profound. For starters, you'll burn more calories. This might lead to weight loss and increased energy. Even better, the muscle activity needed for standing and other movement seems to trigger important processes related to the breakdown of fats and sugars within the body. When you sit, these processes stall — and your health risks increase. When you're standing or actively moving, you kick the processes back into action.

Medications, surgery and other weight strategies

If you're having a hard time losing weight through diet and exercise, you might be wondering what other options are out there.

▶ **Prescription medications.** FDA-approved weight-loss drugs — such as orlistat (Xenical), lorcaserin (Belviq), phentermine (Adipex-P, Suprenza) and phentermine combined with topiramate (Qsymia) — work by reducing your appetite, making you feel full faster, or preventing your body from absorbing fat. These drugs tend to have a number of adverse side effects, and weight loss tends to be moderate. Many individuals regain weight after stopping treatment, and the drugs are intended for use alongside dietary changes and exercise.

▶ **Surgery.** Bariatric surgery refers to a variety of different procedures that are effective for weight loss. It can be a lifesaving surgery for some individuals. It's often used only in adults with severe or complicated obesity. Bariatric surgery does carry a number of risks.

▶ **Complementary and integrative therapies.** Acupuncture has received increasing interest as an alternative weight-loss strategy. Poor study design makes it hard to know whether it's effective, but it may help some women. Other studies have shown stress-relief practices combined with dietary counseling to be effective for weight loss. And though the market for dietary supplements is a staggering $2 billion a year, herbal remedies have very little data supporting their safety and effectiveness for weight loss.

Though these strategies may help some individuals, there's no magic bullet when it comes to achieving and maintaining a healthy weight. The closest thing to it might be establishing long-term healthy habits around diet and exercise.

▶ Set intermediate goals that are SMART: Specific, measurable, attainable, relevant and time-limited. Instead of saying "I'm going to eat better," say "I'm going to eat one more serving of vegetables and fruit each day."

▶ We tend to overestimate our energy expenditure and underestimate our calorie intake. Keeping a food and activity log can help you monitor your habits and is associated with greater weight-loss success. Consider using technology to help you with this. There are numerous wearable devices from manufacturers such as Fitbit, Jawbone, Misfit and more, that help you track your activity levels and the number of calories you burn. Some also monitor your sleep patterns. A wide variety of online and phone apps also are available that help you track your calorie intake and expenditure — *www.loseit.com*, *www.myfitnesspal.com* and *www.my-calorie-counter.com* are just some of the many apps that are out there. A pen and paper also work just fine.

▶ Celebrate your milestones. Treat yourself to a weekend away or a massage. And keep revising your goals as needed.

PRACTICE MINDFULNESS

▶ A holistic approach to weight loss engages the mind as well as the body. Mindfulness — the practice of being attuned to the present moment without judgment — may help you reinforce your positive behaviors.

▶ Tune in to your body and eat when you're hungry. Slow down and enjoy your food, paying attention to the physical sensations and emotions you're feeling as you eat. This gives your body more time to signal that you're full. Eating while your mind is focused elsewhere may lead you to consume more calories, whereas chewing more times before swallowing may help reduce food intake. Stop eating when you're full. Take a pause before you reach for more. You might realize you don't need another serving after all. This more-intuitive approach of noticing and following your body's internal cues has been shown to have positive impacts on healthy habits as well as body image.

▶ Part of weight loss is being able to make healthy decisions in spite of the forces working against you. An increased awareness of your behaviors may help you interrupt your default patterns and choose to engage in actions that are aligned with your goals and values. For example, sometimes you may experience hunger even when you don't physically need food. Being aware of this may help you choose whether to heed these cravings.

▶ Live life to the fullest now, even as you make a commitment to implement healthy changes. Don't wait for the weight to come off to engage in activities you enjoy.

MANAGE YOUR TRIGGERS

▶ Once you're aware of the cues that cause you to eat or avoid exercise, you may be able to circumvent them so that you don't have to rely on your willpower in the moment.

▶ If you eat when you're bored, try distracting yourself with an alternative activity, such as going for a brief walk. If you're always starving after work when you stop to get groceries, consider having a small snack before you leave the office, so you're less tempted to buy unhealthy foods. Create a meal plan and shop for it on the weekend — filling your fridge with fruits and vegetables — so you don't have a "what are we having for dinner tonight?" moment that leads to less healthy choices. Cook healthy dishes on the weekend and freeze or save portions to have during the week.

▶ For many people, TV is a trigger that can affect both diet and exercise, and excessive TV use is associated with an increased risk of obesity and type 2 diabetes. If you're going to watch TV, make it count. Do some strength training or balance exercises during the commercials — or even better, only allow yourself to spend as much time watching TV as you do exercising. And no screen time while eating so that you avoid mindless snacking.

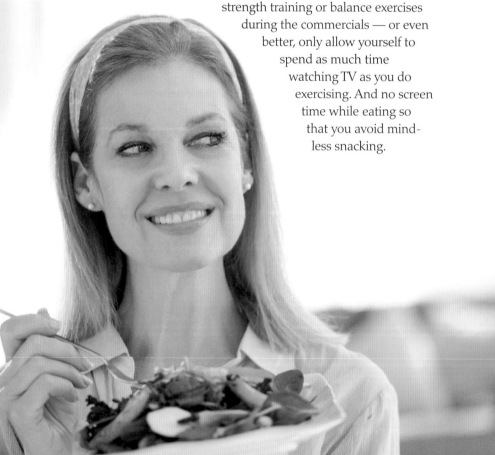

GET SUPPORT

▶ Enlist your spouse, family or friends for support in achieving your weight goals. Let them know specific ways they can help — whether it's exercising with you or just sharing positive encouragement.

▶ Even a canine companion may be a source of motivation and help you stay committed to your regular walks.

▶ Consider signing up for a dedicated weight-loss program or a support group led by a professional.

▶ Remember that you're not alone. Every woman goes through menopause, and though each person's experience is unique, know that many women are likely having the same symptoms and the same struggles with weight management as you are. Just knowing you're all in the same boat may help you keep some perspective as you go through this important life transition.

A worthwhile commitment

This might all seem a bit daunting. You may be juggling a family, a career and an active social life — not to mention dealing with your menopausal symptoms — and now you need to tackle weight loss, too? It's true that — like many worthwhile things — weight management is not necessarily easy. But making a deliberate choice to commit to your health and well-being at this critical time of life is a challenge you can be proud of taking on. Approaching it with a positive attitude can make a big difference in your experience. Your health care provider is also an important source of information and support as you seek to identify weight-related goals and develop strategies to meet them.

CHAPTER TEN

Hormones and other prescription therapies

Perhaps you flipped right to this chapter. Your symptoms are interfering with your life, and you want to get them under control *now*. You've heard that hormone therapy or other prescription drugs might be effective options to get the relief you need. However, you're also concerned about the potential risk if you take these medications. There's a lot of conflicting information out there. How do you sift through all of this information to know what might be the best choice for you?

This chapter will help you understand the different hormonal and nonhormonal prescription therapies available for the treatment of menopausal symptoms and their benefits and risks. Keep in mind, there's s no magic bullet when it comes to treating menopausal symptoms, but after reviewing this chapter you'll be better prepared to have an informed discussion with your health care provider about what treatment may be the most safe and effective for you.

The basic principles on hormones

Hormone therapy is perhaps the most controversial menopause treatment available. And it's true, there's a lot of information to navigate. Before delving into the details, here's a bit of a primer on hormone therapy.

HORMONE THERAPY IS EFFECTIVE There's no question that hormone therapy is the most effective treatment for moderate to severe hot flashes and night sweats, as well as vaginal symptoms that come with menopause, such as dryness, itching, burning and discomfort with intercourse.

THERE ARE BENEFITS AND RISKS Hormone therapy can improve your symptoms and quality of life as you go through this transition, and it may have other health benefits, too. But as with any medication, there also are risks —sometimes significant — that have to be considered. You must evaluate the benefit of therapy in relation to your personal risk.

NOT ALL HORMONE THERAPY TREATMENTS ARE THE SAME It may be tempting to lump all hormonal therapies together and label them as good or bad. But the reality is more complex. There are different treatments available that vary in terms of the hormones used and their dosages, as well as the delivery methods. Each type carries its own benefits and risks. Regardless of the type of hormone therapy, the dosage and duration of treatment should be individualized to your preferences and treatment goals.

HORMONE THERAPY IS NOT RECOMMENDED AS A PREVENTIVE MEAUSURE Hormone therapy has some proven — and some unproven — health benefits beyond treating menopausal symptoms, but it's not recommended for chronic disease prevention or treatment. The exception to this guideline is if you've experienced menopause early. See page 177 for more information on premature menopause and the use of hormone therapy.

THE EXPERTS DO AGREE Given the available information, experts do agree that the benefits of hormone therapy outweigh the risks for healthy women younger than age 60 and within 10 years of their last period who are seeking relief for moderate to severe symptoms of menopause. Although it's not recommended that you start hormone therapy after age 60, continuing treatment past this age may be considered based on your symptoms and risk factors.

With those basics in mind, let's get into the details.

What is hormone therapy?

Hormone therapy is the use of female hormones to treat menopausal symptoms. It was previously referred to as hormone replacement therapy (HRT), but that term has fallen from use as it implies that postmenopausal women are in a deficient state and need to replace lost hormones to achieve a premenopausal level.

After menopause, it's natural to have lower hormone levels and the goal of treatment is not to return them to premenopausal levels but rather to find the lowest effective dose that relieves the symptoms of menopause. Now called hormone therapy (HT), or menopausal hormone therapy, the use of hormones is an effective treatment for symptoms of menopause. The main female sex hormones used in HT include estrogen and a progestogen.

Estrogen is the primary hormone that relieves symptoms of menopause. One of the confusing points about HT is that many of your friends will have different types of therapies prescribed to them. Women are prescribed different types of HT based on whether or not they still have a uterus.

In women who have undergone a hysterectomy and no longer have a uterus, estrogen can be taken alone. This is referred to as estrogen therapy (ET). Women who have not had a hysterectomy need a different approach because giving estrogen alone can cause the lining of the uterus to over-grow. This can lead to precancerous changes and ultimately to cancer of the lining of the uterus (endometrial cancer). To protect the uterine lining from the effects of estrogen and to prevent endometrial cancer, a progestogen is added. This type of treatment with estrogen plus a progestogen is referred to as combination therapy or estrogen-progestogen therapy (EPT).

A bit of history

For over 50 years, millions of women have used hormone therapy to treat their menopausal symptoms. The first hormone therapy preparation — a conjugated estrogen — was first marketed in 1942. Numerous early studies seemed to indicate hormone therapy helped protect women against heart disease, bone loss and dementia. It became widely used both as a treatment for symptoms as well as a preventive health measure. However, over the years, further studies started to cast doubt on some of the reported benefits.

In 1991, the Women's Health Initiative (WHI) was launched. This 15-year nationwide study — which enrolled over 161,000 postmenopausal women — aimed to better understand many common health conditions

Hormone therapy terminology

Here are a few terms that are helpful when learning about hormone therapy.

▶ *Estrogen* is actually a class of many different compounds. The three types produced in the human body are 17beta-estradiol (the most active, or strongest, and the primary estrogen produced by the ovary before meno-pause), estrone (the primary estrogen present in postmenopausal women), and estriol (the form of estrogen produced by the placenta during pregnan-cy). The terms *estradiol* and *17beta-estradiol* refer to the same chemical compound. The term *conjugated estrogens* refers to a combination of numerous estrogens initially derived from pregnant mares' urine. There are also synthetic estrogens, including synthetic conjugated estrogens and ethinyl estradiol (the form of estrogen used in most oral contraceptives).

▶ *Progesterone* is a hormone produced by your ovaries. The same exact chemical compound can be synthetically derived in a laboratory. *Progestins* are synthetic hormones that mimic progesterone but have a different chemical structure. The term *progestogen* refers to any substance with a progesterone-like activity, encompassing both progesterone and progestins.

women experience with age. This was the largest controlled study to date on hormone therapy, and it looked at both estrogen therapy (ET) and estrogen-progestogen therapy (EPT).

The hormone therapy component of WHI was intended to last through 2005, however the EPT arm was stopped in 2002 because of an increased risk of breast cancer in the group taking hormones. Researchers also observed an increased risk of stroke, heart attack and blood clots in this group. The same risks were not initially seen in the ET arm so that arm of the study continued until 2004 when it became apparent that women taking ET without the progestogen were experiencing an increased risk of stroke.

Though both treatments indicated some benefits — a reduced risk of bone fractures with both therapies, a reduced risk of colon cancer with EPT and a slightly reduced risk of breast cancer with ET — these initial results went against the prevailing understanding that hormone therapy had protective effects. The WHI findings were understandably concerning to women and their health care providers and caused an abrupt decline in the use of hormone therapy — as well as much fear and ensuing debate.

WHI results in context

In the years since these initial results were published, the WHI data has continued to be analyzed and reinterpreted, and more studies have been done. This has led the medical community to develop a more nuanced understanding of the risks and benefits of hormone therapy. Some of the initial fears have been allayed, or at least put into context.

For example, though the ages of women participating in the WHI ranged from 50 to 79, the average age was 63 years old — a more advanced age than most women seeking relief from their menopausal symptoms. Some of the women in the study were smokers and had existing heart disease. In addition, the WHI study included just two regimens of hormone therapy — a conjugated equine estrogen alone or in combination with a progestin — in only one dosage delivered by mouth. This is understandable, as the study was designed to examine the most commonly prescribed forms of hormone therapy up to that point. However, we know now that different types of hormones as well as their doses and delivery methods may have different risks for women at different ages (more on that below).

The bottom line — hormone therapy isn't all good or all bad. After a period of widespread use, followed by a time of fear and uncertainty, the pendulum seems to be landing somewhere in the middle. It's understood that hormone therapy does indeed come with some risks, but for many younger healthy women, it's the most effective way to manage menopausal symptoms and improve quality of life.

Who should use — and who should avoid — hormone therapy?

Before answering that question, let's look at what the current evidence seems to be telling us. See pages 172-173 for an overview of some of the health considerations related to hormone therapy.

Overall, study results seem to indicate that hormone therapy poses a greater risk to older women than to younger women. Evidence also indicates that, although it's required to prevent endometrial cancer, the addition of a progestogen to estrogen causes a greater risk of adverse effects than does estrogen alone — although evidence also shows that progesterone may have fewer risks than progestins. In addition, hormones delivered through the skin may have fewer risks than do pills taken orally.

So who should consider taking hormone therapy and who shouldn't?

WHEN YOU MAY WANT TO AVOID HORMONE THERAPY If you have existing cardiovascular disease, a history of blood clots, an already increased risk of stroke, severe liver disease, abnormal vaginal bleeding that hasn't been evaluated, or if you have or have had an estrogen dependent cancer, such as breast or endometrial cancers. Because recent studies indicate that the risk of blood clot and stroke are lower with hormones delivered through the skin as opposed to orally, hormone therapy might be an option for some women at risk of these conditions. Women taking hormone therapy ideally should not smoke. And if menopausal symptoms are mild and not significantly impacting quality of life, hormone therapy isn't needed to stay healthy.

WHEN THE BENEFITS LIKELY OUTWEIGH THE RISKS If you're healthy, under age 60 and within 10 years of your last period, you have moderate to severe menopausal symptoms that are interrupting your sleep or impacting your quality of life, and you don't have specific health conditions that prevent you from using hormone therapy. Also, if you've lost bone mass and you either can't tolerate or aren't benefiting from other treatments to reduce fracture risk, hormone therapy might be a viable option.

To further inform this discussion and help you determine whether hormone therapy is right for you, let's get into the nitty-gritty of the different types of hormone treatments.

Types of hormone therapy

Hormone therapy is available in a number of different delivery methods, preparations and dosages.

DELIVERY METHODS Systemic hormone therapy refers to the delivery of hormones throughout the body to achieve relief of both hot flashes and vaginal symptoms. Systemic hormones can be delivered by mouth (oral delivery), through the skin (transdermal application) with patches, gels or sprays, or with a vaginal ring that delivers a systemic dose of estrogen.

Local therapies affect only one area of the body. In the treatment of menopausal symptoms this means using estrogen to treat vaginal dryness — part of what's known as genitourinary syndrome of menopause. If you're primarily seeking relief from vaginal symptoms and over-the-counter moisturizers and lubricants haven't helped or are not enough, local vaginal estrogen therapy can be delivered by vaginal cream, tablet or ring. The lower doses of hormones used with local vaginal estrogen therapy mean that much less is absorbed into the body, and a progestogen is not needed to protect the uterus. In women with a history of breast cancer, the safety of using these local estrogen treatments for vaginal symptoms is still unproved. Also, if you're taking a low-dose systemic estrogen therapy, you may still need to add local vaginal estrogen therapy in order to address vaginal symptoms.

Your personal preference will influence the delivery method you choose. You may have a hard time swallowing pills, or perhaps you find the cream messy or the adhesive on the skin patch irritating. Other considerations will have more to do with the risks of the various methods. Transdermal delivery methods have generally been shown to have fewer risks than oral — this is likely because hormones absorbed through your skin aren't metabolized by the liver, as are treatments that pass through the digestive tract. However, pills are often less expensive and may still be appropriate for some women. Women using a topical emulsion, gel or spray will need to take precautions to avoid transferring the hormones to children and pets, who can be adversely affected by the exposure. Similarly, vaginal hormone creams shouldn't be used as a lubricant during intercourse. If you are only seeking relief from vaginal symptoms, vaginal estrogen is thought to be the most effective therapy, and you shouldn't need a systemic treatment.

PREPARATIONS As you know by now, hormone treatments for menopausal symptoms will either contain estrogen alone or estrogen plus a progestogen. In perimenopausal women, hormonal contraceptives are often the recommended treatment until you reach menopause, to cover both menopausal symptoms and contraception. Then at the point of menopause, you would switch to a menopausal hormone therapy preparation (see "Contraceptives during the menopausal transition" on page 175).

In the past, the only available hormone preparations were conjugated estrogens and a synthetic progestin. Now there are a variety of other options, including 17beta-estradiol (equivalent to the estrogen produced in your body), synthetic conjugated estrogens, different synthetic progestins and micronized progesterone (equivalent to the progesterone produced in your body). Most of these preparations are available in a variety of delivery methods. Though the different preparations are not inherently better or worse than one another, they may have different risks associated with them. The delivery method also plays a role in the level of risk.

The dosing schedule of hormone therapy depends on a variety of factors. Whereas estrogen therapy is given continuously, the progestogen in combination hormone therapy regimen may be provided either as a continuous regimen — one that's taken daily — or a cyclic regimen, which has periods of treatment interspersed with progestogen-free intervals. There are pros and cons to both continuous and cyclic progestogen. Cyclic dosing may reduce the total days of exposure to progestogens, but it does result in monthly withdrawal bleeding, which can be annoying to many women as one of the benefits of menopause is the end of the menstrual cycle. Taking progestogens continuously leads to amenorrhea in many women — the absence of any monthly bleeding — however, these regimens often cause irregular bleeding, especially the closer to menopause you are. Because progestogen therapy (specifically progesterone) can help with sleep, continuous regimens dosed at bedtime ensure you receive this benefit all of the time, not just for part of the month.

Many women newly into menopause are started on a cyclic regimen — because the risk of breakthrough bleeding is high and scheduled bleeding is often easier to manage than unscheduled bleeding. A change to continuous therapy can then be made once the likelihood of breakthrough bleeding has lessened later on in menopause. However, every woman is different, and other considerations and risk factors will affect the decision regarding what type of dosing regimen is best. If you experience any abnormal vaginal bleeding — especially after a period of amenorrhea — talk to your health care provider right away.

DOSAGE, DURATION AND TRANSITION Most hormone therapy preparations are available in a variety of doses. Experts recommend taking the lowest dose that relieves your symptoms or reaches your treatment goals, and it may take a bit of trial and error to identify this amount. Hormone therapy can have a variety of side effects, including vaginal bleeding, bloating and water retention, breast tenderness, headaches, and mood swings. Using a lower dose may help alleviate these symptoms as well as reduce some of the more-serious risks of hormone therapy. And though many women fear that weight gain is a side effect of hormone therapy, it hasn't been shown to have any effect on weight. And it may reduce your risk of diabetes.

Hormone therapy is generally taken for as long as required to treat symptoms. However, there's no firm cutoff time, and the duration of treatment will be an ongoing conversation between you and your health care provider based on your individual risks, benefits and personal preferences.

Health considerations related to hormone therapy

The hormones you might take to manage menopausal symptoms can affect your body in a variety of ways.

CARDIOVASCULAR DISEASE Accumulating evidence suggests a direct role of the loss of estrogen on the development and progression of atherosclerosis (hardened arteries) — one of the primary causes of cardiovascular disease. This evidence indicates that giving estrogen to younger menopausal women reduces their risk of heart disease.

To describe this relationship, researchers have proposed a "timing hypothesis," which suggests that estrogen therapy has a beneficial effect on cardiovascular health if started soon after menopause, but a detrimental effect if started later. This idea suggests that it's not age per se that determines how estrogen affects the cardiovascular system, but the extent to which atherosclerosis has already developed at the time treatment is started — and older women are likely to have more-advanced atherosclerosis.

BREAST CANCER The relationship is complex. Numerous studies indicate that estrogen-progestogen therapy increases the risk of breast cancer after approximately five years of use. Conversely, recent evidence indicates that estrogen alone does not appear to increase breast cancer risk. However, not all studies have come to this conclusion.

Hormone therapy, particularly estrogen combined with a progestogen, can increase the density of your breasts, making breast cancer more difficult to detect with a mammogram. When it is detected, it may already be at a more advanced stage.

If you have a history of breast cancer, you shouldn't use a systemic hormone treatment, as studies show it is associated with an increased risk of breast cancer recurrence. Local vaginal estrogen can be considered for vaginal symptoms if other treatments haven't worked.

CHOLESTEROL Oral hormone therapies have mixed effects on cholesterol levels. They've been shown to increase levels of high-density lipoprotein ("good") cholesterol and decrease levels of low-density lipoprotein ("bad") cholesterol. Though this is a good thing, they also increase triglyceride levels (not a good thing). Hormone therapies applied to the skin (transdermal therapies) haven't been shown to have these effects.

STROKE Evidence indicates that standard doses of oral hormone therapy can increase the risk of ischemic stroke — where a blood clot travels to the brain and blocks blood flow. For younger postmenopausal women, the absolute risk is quite low, but it's more substantial for older women.

VENOUS THROMBOEMBOLISM Venous thromboembolism (VTE), refers to a blood clot in a deep vein (deep vein thrombosis) or in a lung (pulmonary embolism). Hormone therapy has been shown to increase the risk of VTE. The risk tends to be lower in women who start the treatment early in menopause, and is generally low for younger healthy women. Transdermal treatments also may carry a lower risk of VTE than do oral regimens.

COGNITION The timing hypothesis also may apply here. There is evidence that hormone therapy has a protective effect when used by younger women, and may reduce the risk of Alzheimer's disease. However, it can have a detrimental effect on cognition and dementia in older women.

DIABETES Hormone therapy reduces the risk of diabetes. But as cardiovascular disease is more common in women with diabetes, for women who already have diabetes, it can complicate the assessment of whether hormone therapy is an appropriate treatment option.

OSTEOPOROSIS Estrogen has been shown to prevent and treat bone loss, reducing the risk of fractures. It's approved as a second-choice therapy for the prevention and treatment of osteoporosis.

GALBLADDER DISEASE Hormone therapy may increase the risk of gallstones and gallbladder disease. The risks tend to be greater with oral therapies as opposed to transdermal therapies.

OTHER EFFECTS

▶ **Sleep.** Hormone therapy can help with insomnia and night sweats.

▶ **Mood.** Estrogen may have a positive effect on mood and can help relieve menopause-related mood changes. It seems most effective during perimenopause — when hormone levels are fluctuating.

▶ **Hair.** Hormone therapy may support hair growth.

▶ **Eyes.** Many women experience dry eyes around menopause. Hormone therapy may worsen or improve this condition.

If you and your health care provider decide it's time to transition away from hormone therapy, you'll likely taper off of it, though the research isn't clear that tapering is any better than stopping abruptly when it comes to the recurrence of symptoms. If your symptoms are still moderate to severe after discontinuing treatment, you and your health care provider will decide whether restarting hormone therapy or trying a nonhormonal option is best for you.

PUTTING IT ALL TOGETHER The variety of treatments available today mean that women have many options when it comes to the preparation, delivery method and dose of hormone therapy they take. It may involve a bit of mix and match to find your individualized solution. Some health conditions may help guide your choices, and your personal preference will come into play. The specific treatment that is right for you may change over time.

Alternative options

In addition to standard hormone therapy preparations for menopausal symptoms, other options exist.

TSEC In 2013, the Food and Drug Association (FDA) approved a new type of drug called a tissue-selective estrogen complex (TSEC). This drug pairs a selective estrogen receptor modulator (SERM) with conjugated estrogens. SERMs are estrogen-like compounds but are not hormones per se. As their name implies, they have a selective effect — either blocking or allowing the activity of estrogen in the tissues it acts upon. A number of SERMs are used in the treatment of women's health conditions. For example, the drug raloxifene (Evista) is a SERM used to prevent and treat osteoporosis. Tamoxifen (Soltamox) is used to prevent and treat breast cancer, and ospemifene (Osphena) is used to treat pain during intercourse.

In the case of the TSEC drug Duavee, conjugated estrogens provide relief from hot flashes, and the SERM bazedoxifene is used in place of a progestogen. Bazedoxifene has a protective effect on the uterus, similar to progestogens, but it seems to have a neutral effect on the breasts — not causing the increase in density seen with some progestogens. However, its long-term effect on breast cancer risk is unknown. The drug also reduces the risk of fractures and is approved to prevent osteoporosis.

The TSEC treatment is relatively new, and more research is needed to fully understand its benefits and risks and the role it might play in the treatment of menopausal symptoms. In theory, it offers an alternative to progestogens for women who are concerned about the increased health risks that seem to come from adding a progestogen to estrogen therapy. However, keep in mind that not all progestogens are the same, and evidence indicates that progesterone doesn't seem to have the same adverse effects that have been found with synthetic progestins. In addition, the TSEC pairing still contains oral conjugated estrogens, which are associated with an increased risk of stroke and blood clots.

Contraceptives during the menopausal transition

Combination oral contraceptives containing both estrogen and a progestin are a good option for controlling hot flashes in perimenopausal women who still require birth control. They lead to lighter and more-regular periods — which can be a relief if irregular and heavy bleeding is bothersome. They also help preserve bone density, reduce the risk of ovarian and endometrial cancers, reduce painful cramps, and help manage acne. These combination treatments are generally safe for healthy nonsmokers who aren't overweight, and long-term use hasn't been shown to increase the risk of breast cancer. Progestin-only options can be used in women who smoke or have other health complications that prevent use of a pill containing estrogen; however, the progestin-only treatments likely won't help with hot flashes.

If birth control is your primary goal and you prefer to avoid the hassle of a daily pill, longer term options such as subdermal implants that are inserted just under your skin, a copper IUD or a levonorgestrel-releasing intrauterine system (LNG-IUS) are available. Keep in mind these delivery methods won't improve your hot flashes. The LNG-IUS device is also sometimes used to provide endometrial protection in peri- or postmenopausal women taking estrogen therapy, though it's not approved for this purpose. It can also significantly reduce menstrual bleeding. However, the LNG-IUS may result in systemic absorption of hormones, and more study is needed to determine if this increases breast cancer risk.

Talk with your health care provider about what option is best for you. After menopause, it's recommended that women switch to menopausal hormone therapies as they contain much lower doses of hormones.

BIOIDENTICAL CUSTOM-COMPOUNDED HORMONES When the results of the WHI came out and caused significant concern about the effects of hormone therapy, a number of "bioidentical custom-compounded" treatments popped up that were purported to be safer than commercially available prescriptions. However, this is not necessarily the case, and these treatments should be approached with caution.

What is bioidentical? The term *bioidentical* generally means that the hormones in a product are chemically identical to those your body produces. But this definition is not always used consistently. Marketers of custom-compounded treatments often call their products bioidentical, implying they are more natural than traditional hormone therapies. But a number of FDA-approved estradiol products — such as Estrace, Climara and Vivelle-Dot — are chemically and structurally identical to the compounds made by your body. These are technically "bioidentical," however the FDA chooses not to use this term.

But aren't they custom-made for me? Marketers of custom-compounded hormones say their products are advantageous because they are individualized preparations, made for you based on a blood or saliva test to assess your hormone levels. However, the hormone levels in your saliva or blood can vary greatly from day to day — and even from hour to hour — and don't necessarily reflect the levels in your tissues. In addition, the treatments often attempt to bring every woman's hormones to the same predetermined level. Your symptoms and their severity are a better guide for determining your specific therapy needs.

For these custom treatments, you need to go through a compounding pharmacy — one that specializes in making medications in doses and preparations that are not commercially available. Custom-compounding pharmacies aren't regulated by the FDA, and their products aren't subject to the same rigorous testing and standards for safety, effectiveness, purity and consistency that traditional, commercially available hormonal preparations have to meet. One sampling of bioidentical custom-compounded products conducted by the FDA found that the ingredients varied significantly from what was stated on the label, and the FDA has provided warnings to companies about their misleading marketing claims.

Are they safe? There is no credible scientific data that indicates bioidentical custom-compounded products are safer or more effective than commercially available hormone therapies. They should be presumed to have the same health risks. And the risks may actually be greater with custom-compounded products if the levels of progesterone are not sufficient to protect women from endometrial cancer.

FDA-approved hormone therapies come in a wide variety of options, including a number of products that are identical in structure to those produced by your body. And though you should approach custom-compounded products cautiously, the process is useful in certain circumstances. For example, the commercially available form of micronized progesterone contains peanut oil, so your health care provider may prescribe a custom-compounded version if you have a peanut allergy.

OVER-THE-COUNTER HORMONES You may be curious about using nonprescription hormones and phytoestrogens to treat your symptoms. These products are discussed later in this chapter and in Chapter 11.

Premature menopause and hormone therapy

If you experience premature menopause — whether it occurs naturally or is caused by medical interventions — the early loss of estrogen affects your body in a number of ways. Though premature menopause lowers the risk of breast cancer, it can increase the risk of osteoporosis, heart disease, dementia, sexual dysfunction, mood disorders and even early death.

For women who reach menopause prematurely, the protective benefits of hormone therapy almost always outweigh the risks. Hormone therapy is recommended at least until the average age of menopause (between age 51 and 52 years), at which point you can assess your symptoms, risks and treatment options with your health care provider.

Weighing the benefits and risks

There are a number of factors that play into whether hormone therapy is right for you. You and your health care provider will need to consider:

▶ What symptoms you're experiencing and their severity
▶ Your age
▶ How long it's been since menopause began, or — if you're in perimenopause — whether you still need contraception
▶ Whether or not you have a uterus
▶ Whether you reached menopause naturally or as a result of surgery

- Whether you're experiencing menopause earlier than average
- Your personal history of cancer, especially breast, endometrial and ovarian cancers
- Your family history and risk of cardiovascular disease, blood clots, breast cancer and osteoporosis
- Lifestyle factors, such as your weight and whether you smoke
- Your personal preferences and risk tolerance

REDUCING NEGATIVE EFFECTS If hormone therapy is a good choice for you, here are some ways to reduce the risk of negative effects:

Find the best product and delivery method Talk with your health care provider about the factors listed above to identify what treatment is right for your unique situation.

Minimize the amount you take Work with your health care provider to find the dose that best meets your treatment goals. It may take a bit of trial and error to find the appropriate dose to manage your symptoms. If you're taking hormone therapy because you've experienced early menopause, talk with your health care provider about the dose required to protect your health.

Seek regular follow-up care See your health care provider regularly to ensure that the benefits continue to outweigh the risks and for screenings such as mammograms and cervical cancer screening (see Chapter 17 for more). Make sure to see your health care provider if you experience any unusual vaginal bleeding, especially if you've gone for a period of time with no bleeding.

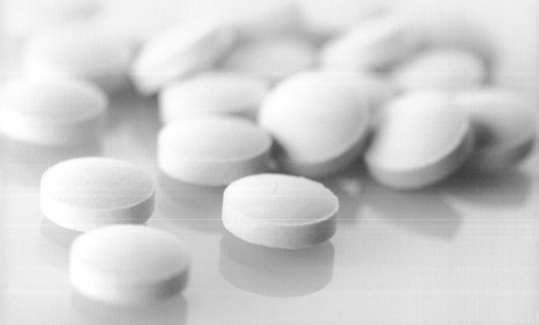

Make healthy lifestyle choices Include physical activity and exercise in your daily routine, eat a healthy diet, maintain a healthy weight, don't smoke, limit alcohol, manage stress, and manage chronic health conditions such as high cholesterol and high blood pressure.

IN PERSPECTIVE Remember that hormone therapy isn't permanent. You can stop your treatment at any point and know that the risks — and also the benefits — will lessen over time.

Though the risks of hormone therapy might scare you off, it's important to keep in mind that all medications and treatments carry a degree of risk. The risks of hormone therapy are actually similar to those seen with other therapeutic treatments that women commonly seek. To put things in perspective — the increased risk of breast cancer associated with combination hormone therapy after five years is about equivalent to the increased risk you'd have from drinking between one and two glasses of wine each day. Though the possible consequences of hormone therapy shouldn't be taken lightly, the benefits usually outweigh the risks for healthy women under age 60 initiating treatment within 10 years of menopause.

Nonhormonal prescription therapies

If you've had breast cancer or other conditions that prevent you from safely using hormone therapy — or you simply find the risks are greater than you're willing to accept — you may be feeling disheartened and wondering what other options are out there for you. Though it's true that hormone therapy is the most effective treatment for hot flashes, there are a number of other options that have also been shown to relieve symptoms.

Lifestyle approaches and complementary medicine may work for some women, and these therapies are discussed further in Chapter 11. There are also a variety of nonhormonal prescription medications available.

LOW-DOSE ANTIDEPRESSANTS Studies have shown that certain selective serotonin reuptake inhibitors (SSRIs) and serotonin and norepinephrine reuptake inhibitors (SNRIs) — typically used as antidepressants — are some of the most effective nonhormonal treatments for hot flashes. These medications may be used if hormone therapy isn't a desirable option. SSRIs and SNRIs may also be a good choice for women who need an antidepressant for a mood disorder in addition to relief from hot flashes, and they are sometimes used alongside hormone therapy for this purpose.

The SSRI paroxetine (Brisdelle) is the first and only nonhormonal prescription treatment approved for treating hot flashes. This treatment is a lower dose (7.5 mg) than what is used for treating mood disorders. Higher doses (10 mg) of paroxetine (Paxil) may be used off-label for menopausal symptoms. Other SSRIs and SNRIs used for hot flashes include escitalopram (Lexapro), citalopram (Celexa), venlafaxine (Effexor XL) and desvenlafaxine (Pristiq).

SSRIs and SNRIs are known to have a range of common side effects, including nausea, dizziness, dry mouth and insomnia. They can also cause sexual problems, such as reduced desire or difficulty with arousal or reaching orgasm — an important consideration if you're already struggling with sexual problems due to menopause. These unpleasant side effects may subside after the first couple weeks of treatment, but some might be persistent. Talk with your health care provider to see if there are ways to minimize these impacts while still getting relief from your hot flashes.

The effectiveness of SSRIs and SNRIs in treating hot flashes can be assessed fairly quickly — generally within two to four weeks. You may need to try a few different SSRIs or SNRIs to see if they are effective for you before deciding to switch to another type of medication. And because the only way to tell whether your symptoms have subsided naturally is to go off of treatment, you'll need to stop taking these medications periodically in order to assess your symptoms.

OTHER MEDICATIONS Antidepressants aren't the only prescription therapies to help with menopausal symptoms. Here are others:

▶ Gabapentin (Neurontin) is a medication used to prevent seizures that has also proved effective in treating hot flashes. The typical treatment requires taking pills three times a day, which some women may find burdensome. Gabapentin has a sedative effect in addition to helping with hot flashes, so it may be a better choice than antidepressants if night sweats are your primary complaint.

▶ Pregabalin (Lyrica) is similar to gabapentin and is used to treat nerve-related pain. Though it seems to be effective in treating hot flashes, it's not been studied as extensively for use in menopausal women.

▶ Clonidine (Catapres) is used to treat high blood pressure and occasionally for menopausal symptoms. However, it's less effective in treating hot flashes than are other medications, and it has unpleasant side effects.

▶ Medications such as eszopiclone (Lunesta), zalepon (Sonata) and zolpidem (Ambien) are used to treat insomnia and have been shown to help improve sleep, though they don't impact hot flashes or night sweats. They may simply help you sleep through the night.

STELLATE GANGLION BLOCK A procedure called stellate ganglion block has shown promise in recent years as a treatment for hot flashes. Typically used for pain relief or to treat excessive sweating, the procedure involves injecting an anesthetic into the stellate ganglion, a group of nerves in the front of your neck. The connection between hot flashes and the stellate ganglion is not quite clear, but the nerves affect blood flow and may influence areas in your brain that regulate body temperature.

The procedure itself takes only a few minutes. It may cause temporary side effects, such as a droopy eyelid on the side of the injection. Stellate ganglion block is generally safe but should be conducted by an experienced practitioner because the injection site is located near arteries, veins and other nerves. The injection can also be costly.

Studies have shown varying levels of effectiveness in using stellate ganglion block to treat hot flashes. A small, randomized clinical trial found that the procedure significantly reduced the frequency and severity of moderate to severe hot flashes, and the results of one injection lasted through the six-month follow-up period. Further research will help health care providers better understand and assess the procedure's effectiveness.

The choice is yours

If you've tried lifestyle modifications and they don't help relieve your symptoms, a prescription therapy — whether hormone-based or not — may be the right choice for you. Given the wide variety of options available, it might take awhile to find the right medication or combination of medications that is effective. This journey may require patience — and a good fan in your bedroom — as you refine your treatment plan.

Whatever option you choose, it's important to keep in touch with your health care provider. Researchers continue to learn more, and new medications may become available. And keep in mind that the best treatment for you may change over time. You'll need to reassess the risks and benefits of different therapies as you age and as your symptoms evolve.

CHAPTER ELEVEN

Complementary and integrative medicine

Perhaps you have a renewed interest in your overall health and wellness during this midlife transition. Or maybe you're looking for alternatives to hormone therapy, prescription medications and other conventional strategies for your menopausal symptoms. Whatever the reason, you've ventured into the world of integrative medicine, formerly called complementary and alternative medicine (CAM).

Integrative medicine refers to a variety of health approaches expanding beyond Western mainstream medicine. Many integrative medicine modalities are based in traditional healing practices, sometimes being centuries to millennia old. They focus away from disease management and to healing, holistic care. Integrative treatments are increasingly being used alongside conventional practices, and research continues to evaluate these approaches. It's estimated that up to 60 percent of Americans use some form of complementary and integrative medicine.

   Some complementary health approaches and products may alleviate common menopausal symptoms. Others may have applications for treating additional conditions women experience in midlife. While this chapter doesn't provide an exhaustive list of integrative therapies, it will cover some popular products and practices you may be considering.

If you choose to try integrative treatments, you should know that the scientific evidence for their effectiveness is often weaker than that for pharmaceutical interventions. They are generally considered less effective than hormone therapy for treating menopausal symptoms. Some alternative approaches may provide an adequate degree of relief in women with mild to moderate symptoms. However, the safety of integrative therapies should not be assumed, and some have the potential for serious side effects or interactions with medications. Make sure to discuss your plans ahead of time with your health care provider.

Mind-body practices

Mind-body practices rely on the connection between mind and body to promote health and wellness. Although they don't necessarily target the hormonal fluctuations of menopause directly, they can relieve stress, improve mood and sleep patterns, and increase quality of life and your ability to cope with this life transition. They are generally low risk and safe to try, and many adults are turning to these practices for relaxation and well-being.

YOGA Originating in India, over 20 million Americans now practice this combination of physical postures, controlled breathing and meditation.

Yoga is associated with a number of health benefits. It may help relieve pain, reduce your heart rate and blood pressure, relieve anxiety and depression, improve sleep, reduce stress, and generally improve your quality of life. It can also improve strength, balance and flexibility, though it has less effect on aerobic fitness. Some studies have shown that mind-body practices like yoga, tai chi and qi gong may improve hot flash symptoms to a similar and possibly greater extent than do more traditional types of physical activity.

Practicing safely

Movement-based techniques, while generally gentle, do have a small risk of injury if not done properly. Find a reputable instructor who can show you how to carry out the movements correctly and safely. These practices should never be painful — begin with comfortable movements and build to more advanced work. These techniques can be done alone or in a group setting. Check your community for classes or providers.

TAI CHI Originating as a form of martial arts in China, tai chi (TIE-CHEE) also has benefits as a health and wellness practice. It's a series of gentle, flowing, movements combined with focused breathing and awareness. It's said to help facilitate the flow of qi (chee) — or vital energy — in the body. Tai chi is practiced for a variety of health benefits, including improved balance, coordination, strength and sleep, and more research is needed to understand its potential benefits.

QI GONG Part of traditional Chinese medicine, the practice of qi gong (CHEE-gung) incorporates meditation, physical movement and breathing exercises to restore and maintain balance. Some evidence indicates that qi gong may improve sleep for women experiencing menopause-related sleep disturbances, as well as vasomotor symptoms.

COGNITIVE BEHAVIORAL THERAPY Also known as CBT, cognitive behavioral therapy is a type of mental health counseling, or psycho-therapy. CBT explores the connection between thoughts, feelings and behaviors, and may be a helpful treatment for menopausal symptoms in some women.

Through self-observation, CBT helps people identify inaccurate or unhealthy beliefs and then reframe them into more constructive thoughts. It's been shown to be effective in treating depression and anxiety, and can be an effective tool for learning how to more effectively manage stressful life situations.

Some studies have shown that both individual and group CBT may help with the management of hot flashes and night sweats. It's likely that the therapy reduces the perception and impact of hot flashes — perhaps by reducing anxiety and providing an increased sense of control — rather than reducing the actual frequency or severity of hot flashes. CBT is generally safe and is a widely used type of therapy.

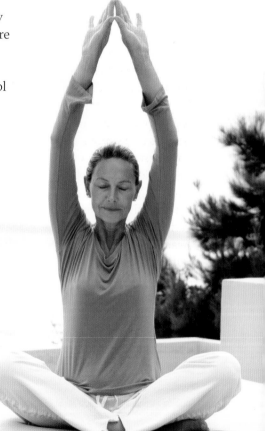

PACED BREATHING A type of deep, rhythmic breathing, paced breathing is intended to promote relaxation by reducing the levels of stress chemicals produced by your body. It may be a helpful practice to try when you start to experience a hot flash. See pages 76-77 in Chapter 4 for a detailed overview of paced breathing.

MEDITATION Meditation is an inexpensive and safe mind-body technique that has been practiced for thousands of years. It's often used to reduce stress and create a relaxed state. Research suggests it may have many additional health benefits, such as reducing blood pressure and relieving anxiety, depression and insomnia. There are many different types of meditation you can try. Most involve eliminating outside distractions, focusing your attention and adopting a nonjudgmental mindset. Some research has shown that mindfulness-based practices may help reduce the impact of hot flashes.

Other integrative approaches

In addition to mind-body techniques, there are a variety of other practices that take a holistic approach to health and wellness.

ENERGY THERAPIES A number of complementary medicine practices are based on the idea that natural energy fields can be balanced or adjusted to foster health. These include practices such as acupuncture, reiki, healing touch and magnetic therapy. Acupuncture is probably the most well-known energy therapy. Originating in China over 2,000 years ago, it's now widely practiced in the U.S. Acupuncture involves the insertion of very thin needles into your skin at specific points in the body. Though researchers are still studying how and why acupuncture might have beneficial effects, in traditional Chinese medicine the practice is said to rebalance the body's vital energy (qi).

Research indicates that acupuncture can help relieve pain related to a variety of conditions, and it may prevent or reduce the frequency of headaches. Some studies suggest acupuncture may reduce hot flashes and improve sleep and mental health in menopausal women, but the studies are generally small and are difficult to combine into large meta-analyses given the individual nature of the therapy. Still, some have shown benefit.

Acupuncture is generally low risk when practiced by a competent, certified practitioner who uses sterile, disposable needles. You may experience some soreness, minor bleeding or bruising at the needle site.

MANUAL THERAPIES Manual, or hands-on, therapies refer to techniques that involve applying physical touch to the body in order to improve symptoms and promote health. If you've ever had a massage, you've already tried a hands-on therapy. And though it may seem like a luxury, massage has therapeutic benefits. With a well-trained provider, massage may relieve pain, reduce anxiety and depression, foster relaxation, and improve sleep — all results you may be seeking as you go through menopause. There are a variety of massage styles, ranging from gentle strokes to deep manipulation of your muscles.

Manipulative therapy — commonly practiced by chiropractors and osteopathic doctors — may be another familiar approach. It involves the application of controlled force to a muscle or joint to relieve symptoms. Other hands-on therapies include the Feldenkrais method and the Alexander technique, which foster a heightened awareness of your posture and your body movements (although they haven't been studied specifically in menopause).

Though hands-on treatments are generally safe when practiced by an experienced and certified or licensed practitioner, women with certain health conditions may need to avoid these therapies. Talk with your health care provider to find out if you need to take precautions.

AYURVEDA Translated as "the science of life" in Sanskrit, ayurveda is a healing system that originated in India. It takes an integrated approach, combining practices such as yoga and massage with nutrition interventions, including herbal remedies and detoxification. There are few studies of the effects of ayurvedic practices on menopausal symptoms, but some women may find the approach or its individual components helpful.

TRADITIONAL CHINESE MEDICINE (TCM) Chinese herbal and dietary therapies have been studied for relief of menopausal symptoms. Most research is inconclusive or conflicting. A small number of studies suggested TCM therapies were effective at improving mood and sleep and reducing hot flashes — though less effective than standard hormone therapy. Some of the individual herbal supplements used in this complex practice are discussed later in this chapter.

Another concept of TCM is the balance of yin and yang. Chinese dietary therapy incorporates high yin (cooling) foods such as cucumber and melon in the management of hot flashes. Women with hot flashes are often encouraged to avoid spicy foods — as they may trigger hot flashes — so there's little harm in trying this method.

Vitamins and minerals

With a renewed focus on your health in midlife, you might be wondering if you're getting adequate vitamins and minerals or have a deficiency.

Vitamins and minerals are micronutrients essential to your body's functioning. They support a variety of internal processes — including building strong bones and teeth, supporting healthy skin and vision, promoting immune system functioning, and much more. Ensuring you're getting enough — but not too much — of these compounds can help you maximize your nutrition and health.

Calcium and vitamin D

Both calcium and vitamin D play an important role in maintaining bone health as you age. Getting the recommended daily amounts is critical early in life to optimize peak bone density, but is also important around the time of menopause, when bone thinning becomes a more immediate concern.

See Chapter 13 for more information on the importance of calcium and vitamin D for bone health.

EAT YOUR GREENS Vitamins and minerals are found in a variety of foods, especially whole, plant-based foods. Although diets high in fruits and vegetables have been associated with a reduced risk of disease, it's unclear if taking a multivitamin or dietary supplement promotes health or prevents disease. Additionally, many vitamins and supplements have associated risks.

It's preferable to get vitamins and minerals from dietary sources. If you're eating a healthy, varied and balanced diet as discussed in Chapter 9, you're probably meeting your nutritional needs and don't need a multivitamin. If your diet is restricted, or if you have issues with digestion and absorption, then you may need a supplement to support your intake. Your health care provider can help you determine whether vitamin or mineral supplements are a good choice for you.

With any supplement, watch out for too much of a good thing. Vitamins that are fat-soluble — that is, they dissolve in fat — are stored in your body for a long time. They may have a greater potential to build up in your system. Fat-soluble vitamins include A, D, E and K.

Vitamins	Recommended daily intake for women ages 31-70
Vitamin A	700 micrograms (mcg)
Vitamin B-1 (thiamin)	1.1 milligrams (mg)
Vitamin B-2 (riboflavin)	1.1 mg
Vitamin B-3 (niacin)	14 mg
Vitamin B-6 (pyridoxine)	1.3 mg (ages 31-50) 1.5 mg (ages 51-70)
Vitamin B-9 (folate, folic acid)	400 mcg
Vitamin B-12 (cyanocobalamin)	2.4 mcg
Vitamin C	75 mg 110 mg (smokers)
Vitamin D	600 international units (IU) (800 IU for women over 70)*
Vitamin E	15 mg or 22.5 IU
Vitamin K	90 mcg[†]

Minerals	
Calcium	1,000 mg (ages 31-50) 1,200 mg (ages 51-70)
Chromium	25 mcg (ages 31-50)[†] 20 mcg (ages 51-70)[†]
Copper	900 mcg
Iron	18 mg (ages 31-50) 8 mg (ages 51-70)
Magnesium	320 mg
Manganese	1.8 mg[†]
Molybdenum	45 mcg
Phosphorus	700 mg
Selenium	55 mcg
Zinc	8 mg

Source: Dietary Reference Intakes. Institute of Medicine.

*The National Osteoporosis Foundation recommends 400 to 800 IU of vitamin D a day for women under age 50 and 800 – 1,000 IU for women age 50 and older.

†Adequate intake — no established daily recommended intake.

HOW MUCH DO YOU NEED? A balanced approach is required when it comes to vitamins and minerals. Too much of some may block the absorption of others or result in adverse effects. And yet certain vitamins or minerals — in the right amounts — are needed to facilitate the uptake of others.

Thankfully, there are established guidelines known as Dietary Reference Intakes (DRIs) to help you determine a healthy range for micronutrient needs — see the table on page 188. The standards are based on general age ranges for the average population, so talk with your health care provider to find out if your own needs might differ.

The units used for each vitamin or mineral may vary slightly — for example, some are measured in milligrams (mg) or micrograms (mcg) and others in international units (IU). Though this might get confusing, most supplements will tell you what percentage of the recommended daily intake is provided. You may have to ask your health care provider or search a reputable website to find out how much is contained in dietary sources, especially if you're eating whole foods that don't come with a nutrition label. The U.S. Department of Agriculture's SuperTracker resource — *www.supertracker.usda.gov* — allows you to look up the nutrition information for a wide variety of foods. Keep in mind that the recommended daily levels for vitamins and minerals refer to intake from all sources.

Alternatives for hot flashes

Many women are interested to know whether over-the-counter hormones or other supplements might be useful to help relieve hot flashes. They might, but conclusive evidence is usually limited or conflicting.

TOPICAL PROGESTERONE Numerous creams and gels are available that contain progesterone. These products are often made from soybeans or wild yam. They are promoted to have many anti-aging health benefits beyond treating menopausal symptoms.

Progesterone creams are relatively safe, and studies have shown they may provide some degree of hot flash relief. However, because dosages and concentrations are inconsistent, the actual absorption of progesterone varies and these creams most likely do not provide enough of the hormone for uterine protection. They shouldn't be used for this purpose. Some wild yam creams are specifically marketed to contain a compound called diosgenin, which is advertised as a precursor to progesterone. However, your body can't actually convert this ingredient to progesterone.

PHYTOESTROGENS AND ISOFLAVONES If you've been searching for relief from your hot flashes, you've probably heard of phytoestrogens and isoflavones. Phytoestrogens are a variety of plant-based compounds that have weak estrogen-like properties.

Isoflavones are one type of phytoestrogen and have been the most studied for use in treating menopausal symptoms. They're found in legumes such as soybeans, lentils, chickpeas and beans. Soy products contain the highest levels of isoflavones and thus have received the most attention.

Soy Many studies on the impact of soy isoflavones on hot flashes have been inconclusive. However, there's an emerging understanding that — although not as effective as hormone therapy — soy-derived isoflavones can modestly improve hot flashes and quality of life for postmenopausal women. And, though isoflavones haven't generally been found to improve vaginal symptoms of menopause, some research has indicated that an isoflavone-based topical gel may help treat vaginal dryness.

Recent studies have helped researchers better understand the specific types of isoflavones that may be most beneficial for hot flashes and other health conditions. Hot flash improvement related to soy intake seems to be related to two specific isoflavones — genistein and daidzein.

When daidzein is broken down by your intestinal bacteria, it produces a compound called equol. Equol has estrogen-like effects on the body that may help with menopausal symptoms. Only some women have the bacteria necessary to produce equol — it's estimated that 25 to 35 percent of North American women are equol producers, compared with as many as 60 percent of women in Asian countries.

In general, studies haven't found isoflavones to be effective in preventing bone loss or conveying cognitive benefits. However, some initial evidence indicates that equol producers who consume dietary soy may see greater benefits in these realms — as well as with hot flash control — compared with nonequol producers. With regard to cardiovascular benefits, soy isoflavones likely have a minimal impact on lowering cholesterol and blood pressure, though they might help your arteries retain flexibility. As with the use of prescription hormone therapy, there is a timing hypothesis at play, suggesting that this beneficial effect may be seen if soy is used early on after menopause. A woman's equol-producing status may also affect whether or not she experiences these cardiovascular benefits.

There's a lot more to learn about the effectiveness and long-term safety of equol and other soy isoflavones. Currently, there's no commercially available test you can take to determine whether or not you produce equol. The low number of equol producers in the U.S. means that soy products may not

Isoflavones and cancer risk

Because isoflavones have estrogen-like effects, their safety with regard to breast and endometrial cancers has been examined. So far, research suggests dietary soy doesn't increase the risk of breast or endometrial cancer. In some studies, soy intake was associated with a slightly reduced risk of breast cancer. This was primarily in Asian women, indicating that equol production may play a role. Soy hasn't been associated with an increased risk of breast cancer recurrence, and dietary soy is likely safe for breast cancer survivors. However, women with breast cancer should generally avoid soy supplements until more information is available about their long-term safety.

give you much relief from your symptoms, and concentrated soy supplements should be approached with caution. For most women, though, there's little harm in including whole soy foods as part of a balanced diet.

Red clover Red clover also belongs to the legume plant family and is a source of isoflavones. A number of studies have shown that red clover supplements are not effective in relieving menopausal symptoms. Though red clover seems safe for short-term use, there's a lack of safety evidence for long-term use and in women with a history of hormone-dependent cancers.

BOTANICAL SUPPLEMENTS In addition to phytoestrogens, there are a number of other plant-based supplements that are sought for hot flash relief.

Black cohosh A member of the buttercup family, the black cohosh plant has been used in Europe for many years to treat menopausal symptoms. It may help manage hot flashes and, when combined with St. John's wort, improve mood. There's limited evidence supporting its effectiveness, but it may work for some women. Black cohosh doesn't seem to have estrogen-like effects, as was originally thought, though it may interfere with the effectiveness of tamoxifen. There have also been concerns about a potential association between black cohosh and liver failure. If you take black cohosh, make sure you find a high-quality supplement and talk to your health care provider if you experience any symptoms of a liver reaction, such as yellow skin, loss of appetite, dark urine or severe abdominal pain.

Evening primrose oil Native to North America, the seeds of the evening primrose plant contain gamma-linoleic acid, an essential fatty acid. Supplements are promoted for hot flash relief, but there's little scientific evidence to support their effectiveness for this or other uses. Though evening prim-rose oil is well-tolerated by many people, it can also have a number of adverse side effects, including, diarrhea, blood clots, reduced immune system functioning and seizures in women taking antipsychotic medication. It shouldn't be used with blood thinners or antipsychotic drugs.

Sage The common garden herb you may be familiar with for culinary uses is also a traditional folk remedy. Some women use it to treat hot flashes. Small studies have shown some effectiveness, but evidence is limited. Sage is generally safe, but avoid oil-based preparations, as they contain a compound called thujone, which affects the nervous system. It may cause vomiting, seizures, kidney damage and dizziness.

Hypnosis for hot flashes?

You may be willing to try almost anything to manage your hot flashes. Accumulating evidence suggests that hypnosis might be one of few nonpharmaceutical treatments that are truly effective for hot flash control.

Though one trial found that hypnosis helped reduce the frequency and severity of hot flashes, data is limited. More studies are needed to estab-lish its effectiveness in treating menopausal symptoms.

Other common supplements

In addition to hot flash relief, you may be seeking alternative approaches for other health concerns. Many of the treatments below have long been used in medicinal preparations; however, conclusive scientific data on their effectiveness and long-term safety is often lacking.

FOR MOOD

Ginseng Some evidence suggests that the root of the Asian *Panax ginseng* plant — a mainstay of Chinese medicine — may help improve well-being and mood, but not hot flashes. Short-term use at recommended doses seems safe, and further study is needed to assess long-term safety. Be aware that ginseng may lower blood sugar levels and increase blood pressure. It may also increase uterine bleeding, so use caution if you're taking an anticoagulant.

Kava Kava, a member of the pepper family, is native to the South Pacific islands. Research has shown kava supplements to be effective in reducing anxiety, though its impact on hot flashes is inconclusive. Kava use has been associated with cases of liver failure and hepatitis, and the supplement is banned in some countries. Kava may also cause drowsiness and muscle spasms, and it can interact with other drugs. Consult with your health care provider before using kava.

S-adenosylmethionine (SAM-e) Though evidence is inconclusive, some research indicates SAM-e may be effective in relieving mild to moderate depression. See more information on this supplement in the joint health section on page 197.

St. John's wort The flowers of this herb have been used for centuries in medicinal preparations. Some research indicates St. John's wort is effective in treating mild to moderate depression. It's also been used to treat hot flashes, either on its own or alongside black cohosh. St. John's wort can interact with numerous drugs, including immunosuppressants, antidepressants, contraceptives, cancer treatment drugs and anticoagulants. It may reduce the effectiveness of tamoxifen. If you are taking other medications, talk with your health care provider or pharmacist before trying St. John's wort.

Valerian The valerian plant has long been used as a medicinal plant in Europe. Supplements are made from its roots and underground stems. Valerian has shown some effectiveness in reducing anxiety, but needs more study. It has few side effects with short-term use, but its long-term safety hasn't been established.

Vitex The fruit of the shrublike vitex tree has been used to treat menstrual symptoms for thousands of years. Though reliable evidence is lacking, supplements may help perimenopausal women manage PMS and irregular bleeding. Vitex is not known to cause serious side effects, though it may negatively affect sexual desire. This has earned the plant its common name — chasteberry. Vitex may also increase the likelihood of pregnancy. Vitex shouldn't be used alongside antipsychotic medications or those used to treat Parkinson's disease, as it may affect dopamine levels in the brain.

FOR SLEEP

Melatonin The hormone melatonin plays a role in your body's natural sleep-wake cycle. Research results on the effectiveness of melatonin supplements are mixed, and there is limited evidence to show they provide relief from menopause-related sleep issues. Melatonin supplements may be most effective when treating sleep issues related to circadian rhythm disturbances, such as shift work or jet lag. They are generally safe for short-term use,

Supplement safety

A vast world of products fall under the umbrella of dietary supplements. Some supplements can be part of a healthy lifestyle and are safe in recommended doses, while others have significant safety concerns. It's always good to assess supplements with a critical eye.

Keep in mind that supplements — like prescription medications — can affect your body in many ways. They may have side effects that range from mildly bothersome to potentially life-threatening. And, they can have harmful interactions with other supplements, prescription medications and over-the-counter drugs. Many supplements need more scientific study before their effectiveness and safety are established.

Dietary supplements are governed by different rules from those that apply to prescription drugs. Supplements don't go through the same rigorous testing and approval process to establish their safety and effectiveness. It's up to each manufacturer to ensure that product labeling is sufficient and truthful, and that the product is safe and effective. Labels might not contain information about adverse effects or possible drug interactions. And though the Food and Drug Administration (FDA) can monitor products once they are on the market, it has little power to step in until after a concern is brought to light.

Some companies do make high-quality products. But it can be challenging to separate the good from the bad. Here are some tips that will help you approach supplements safely:

though the safest dose for long-term use isn't known. High doses are associated with a range of adverse effects and can worsen depression.

Valerian Though it needs more study, valerian may help improve sleep and is a traditional remedy for insomnia. Valerian is discussed in greater detail in the section on mood (pages 192-193).

FOR MEMORY

Ginkgo Ginkgo seeds and leaf extracts have been used in Chinese medicine for thousands of years to treat a variety of ailments. Supplements are primarily promoted for their cognitive benefits, however research results are generally mixed and the evidence is unreliable. There are some reports of allergic reactions to ginkgo, and the seeds should be avoided due to toxicity concerns. It may cause bleeding, so use caution if you're taking anticoagu-

- Avoid self-prescribing supplements. If you're getting information online, make sure it's from a trusted source and discuss it with your health care provider.

- Look for products labeled with U.S. Pharmacopeial Convention (USP) seal, which generally indicates good quality control. Others used include good manufacturing practices (GMPs), or NSF International.

- Don't assume something marketed as "natural" means it's safe. Many natural compounds are poisonous to humans.

- Be wary of products claiming immediate or drastic effects. If it sounds too good to be true, it probably is.

- Avoid "more is better" thinking. Even compounds your body requires, such as vitamins and minerals, can be toxic in high doses. And, you might waste money on unnecessary products.

- If you're taking supplements or drugs, keep good track of the amount you take, how frequently you take it and any side effects you experience.

- Discuss your needs and questions with your health care provider or pharmacist before taking any supplements. Both can help you navigate the options available as you seek to optimize your health and wellness.

lants. Animal studies have shown tumor development with long-term use, and more study is needed to know if ginkgo affects cancer risk in humans.

Ginseng Traditionally used to improve mental performance, Asian ginseng has been studied for use in treating Alzheimer's disease. However, research results are inconclusive. See the section on mood (pages 192-193) for more information on ginseng's use for sleep and mood concerns.

FOR CARDIOVASCULAR HEALTH

Coenzyme Q10 Coenzyme Q10 (CoQ10) is an antioxidant found in the human body and elsewhere in nature. It's necessary for proper cell functioning, and low natural levels have been associated with a variety of diseases. CoQ10 may benefit some women with cardiovascular conditions such as congestive heart failure. More research is needed to determine its effectiveness in treating other health concerns. CoQ10 is relatively safe, though it may interfere with chemotherapy. Some side effects include insomnia, rashes, nausea, dizziness, heartburn and headaches.

Fish oil Fish oil has become a popular supplement because it contains omega-3 fatty acids — polyunsaturated fats that are thought to provide a wide range of health benefits. Fish oil has been found to have cardiovascular benefits — lowering triglyceride levels and blood pressure. A prescription form (Lovaza) is available to treat very high triglyceride levels. Omega-3s from fish oils may help relieve pain from rheumatoid arthritis, and more research is being done on the possible benefits fish oil and omega-3s may have for cognitive health, depression and other conditions. Fish oil is generally safe, though it may cause indigestion, diarrhea and fishy-smelling breath. It can slow blood clotting, and supplements should be used with care if you're taking an anticoagulant. Keep in mind that you can also get fish oil through your diet by eating fatty fish — such as salmon, mackerel, sardines and herring — and shellfish.

DHEA supplements

Dehydroepiandrosterone (DHEA) is a natural substance produced by your adrenal gland and ovaries that your body then turns into estrogen and testosterone. It can also be purchased as a dietary supplement. It's a type of male sex hormone (androgen), though it's also found in women, albeit in lower amounts. DHEA levels decline gradually with age.

DHEA supplements are promoted for anti-aging properties and for boosting sexual desire. There's also interest in their use for improving well-being and cognition and for reducing bone loss. This may make it an appealing product around the time of menopause. However, there is a lack of evidence supporting its use, as well as concerns about harmful side effects. The long-term health impacts and risks for women are unknown.

Some evidence suggests that vaginal preparations of DHEA may be effective for treating vaginal dryness. Preparations absorbed through the skin also are of interest. There are currently no prescription androgen products specifically designed for women, and more research is needed on the potential use of DHEA in treating female health concerns.

If you're trying to bolster your sexual arousal, make sure you've identified and treated any other potential causes — such as vaginal dryness, stress or anxiety — before trying DHEA. See Chapter 7 for more information on sexual health during menopause.

Red yeast rice A fermented rice product, red yeast rice contains a compound called monacolin K. This compound has the same chemical structure as lovastatin, a common statin drug used to treat high cholesterol. Supplements with high amounts of monacolin K have been shown to reduce cholesterol levels. However, the FDA has determined that red yeast rice products containing anything more than trace amounts of monacolin K can't be sold as over-the-counter supplements.

As with most dietary supplements, the quantity of active ingredient can vary greatly and labels often don't show the monacolin K content. Similar to prescription statins, muscular pain and weakness are potential side effects. More study is needed to determine the safety of red yeast rice. If you're concerned about your cholesterol levels, talk with your health care provider about treatment options.

FOR JOINT HEALTH

Glucosamine and chondroitin Glucosamine and chondroitin are natural compounds found in your cartilage tissue. Supplements have been studied for their use in treating joint pain related to osteoarthritis; however, results are mixed as to whether they are helpful for this purpose. Glucosamine and chondroitin supplements are generally safe with few side effects, though glucosamine can enhance the effects of anticoagulants. Glucosamine supplements are made from the skeletons of shellfish, so women with shellfish allergy should use with caution.

S-adenosylmethionine Also called SAM-e, S-adenosylmethionine is produced in the human body from the amino acid methionine. SAM-e plays a role in numerous body functions. It may be useful for treating depression, alleviating pain related to osteoarthritis, and preventing liver disease, but more study is needed to establish its effectiveness. SAM-e was found to be safe with few side effects during short-term use, though longer term safety information — including drug interactions — isn't yet known.

An alternative approach

Though complementary and integrative health treatments may not be as effective as hormone therapy in alleviating common menopausal symptoms, they might bring you a degree of relief and can provide much-needed options for some women. Just remember the safety tips in this chapter and be a discerning consumer. These treatment options can be part of the ongoing conversation you have with your health care provider.

PART FOUR

Health in menopause and beyond

CHAPTER TWELVE

Caring for your breasts

Regardless of how you feel about your breasts, they've been a part of your physical experience as a woman from the early stages of puberty through today. From a biological perspective, breasts are for feeding babies; but they are intertwined in a woman's sexual, physical and emotional experiences as well. For some women, their breasts are a source of pride; for others, breasts may evoke feelings of embarrassment, discomfort, inconvenience or fear. A woman's perception of her breasts may be complex and change through different phases of her life. All women, however, will experience physical changes in their breasts over time.

Perimenopause and menopause are associated with significant changes in your breasts, and mark a time when monitoring your breast health becomes more important. In particular, in the years leading up to menopause, you and your health care provider will discuss breast cancer screening options. The American Cancer Society reports that a woman living in the U.S. has a 1 in 8 lifetime risk of being diagnosed with breast cancer. This means that given the current rates of breast cancer, 1 in 8 women living today will develop breast cancer before the age of 85.

But what are *your* risks of developing the disease and how does *your* risk change over time? Is there anything you can do to reduce that risk? What screening options are best for you and with what frequency? This chapter will help you sort out these questions.

A look inside

Breasts are composed mainly of connective and fatty tissues. Suspended within the tissues of each breast is a network of milk-forming lobes. Within each lobe are many smaller lobules, each of which ends in dozens of tiny bulbs that can produce milk. Thin tubes called ducts connect the bulbs, lobules and lobes to the nipple, which is surrounded by an area of dark skin, called the areola. No muscles are in the breasts themselves, but the chest wall muscles covering your ribs lie underneath each breast.

Blood vessels and lymph vessels run throughout your breasts. Blood nourishes breast cells. Lymph vessels carry a clear fluid called lymph, which contains immune system cells and drains waste products from tissues. Lymph vessels lead to pea-sized collections of tissue called lymph nodes. Most of the lymph vessels in the breast lead to lymph nodes under the arm, called axillary lymph nodes.

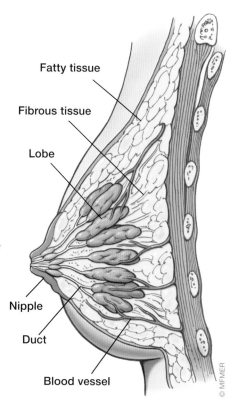

Fatty tissue

Fibrous tissue

Lobe

Nipple

Duct

Blood vessel

© MFMER

CHANGES WITH MENOPAUSE The changes in your breasts during perimenopause and menopause are the result of hormonal changes that occur during this time. During perimenopause, you may notice at times that your breasts become more tender and swollen as estrogen levels fluctuate significantly. Later, as you approach menopause and estrogen levels decrease, the texture, shape and size of your breasts may also change.

You may notice a bumpy texture or lumpiness in your breasts, along with swelling, tenderness or pain. These are known as fibrocystic changes. While fibrocystic changes are common in menstruating women just before their periods, they can also occur in postmenopausal women taking hormone therapy. Menopausal hormone therapy may also make your breasts become more dense than they would otherwise be.

WHAT ABOUT CANCER? Cancer occurs when some cells begin growing abnormally. These cells divide more rapidly than healthy cells do and continue to accumulate, forming a lump or mass.

Breast cancer is the common term for a cancerous (malignant) tumor that starts in cells that line the ducts and lobules of the breast. If the cancer cells are confined to the ducts or lobules and haven't invaded surrounding tissue, the cancer is called *noninvasive.* Cancer that has spread through the walls of the ducts or lobules into connective or fatty tissue is referred to as *invasive.* Cancerous cells may spread (metastasize) through your breast to your lymph nodes or to other parts of your body.

The starting point matters. When abnormal cells are confined within the walls of the duct, this is known as ductal carcinoma *in situ* (DCIS). This condition may progress to invasive cancer over time and is therefore treated as breast cancer. Lobular carcinoma *in situ* (LCIS), in contrast, is not considered a breast cancer because the abnormal cells within the lobules don't usually progress to invasive cancer. However, women with LCIS are still at increased future risk of developing breast cancer.

Breast cancer is the most common life-threatening cancer to affect women worldwide. Until scientists find a way to prevent breast cancer, the best way to fight the disease remains the same — to find it as early as possible.

Breast cancer screening

You shouldn't be worried if your health care provider has suggested that you begin breast cancer screening. The purpose of screening is to detect disease, such as cancer, in its earliest stages when it's the most responsive to treatment. Early detection of breast cancer reduces the need for aggressive treatment options and increases the chance of a cure.

There are a variety of breast cancer screening tests that may be used. The screening methods your health care provider recommends will be based on your breast cancer risk factors. For women at average risk, the screening technique that's universally recommended is mammography. Some organizations also recommend clinical breast examinations — although this practice has come into question in recent years.

MAMMOGRAPHY Mammography is an X-ray examination used to screen for breast cancer or to evaluate abnormalities noted on the breast examination. Low doses of radiation are used to create detailed images of the breasts. These images are captured on film or digitally stored on a computer. From these images, a radiologist can detect changes in breast tissue or evaluate areas of concern.

A screening mammogram is a breast X-ray that's done to detect breast cancer in a person with no breast symptoms or abormality. A diagnostic mammogram is a breast X-ray used to investigate changes in the breast such as a lump, new onset differences in the size or shape of your breasts, nipple discharge or a thickening of a nipple, or change in the texture of the breast tissue. The diagnostic mammogram may involve additional testing such as spot compression images taken to magnify an area of concern in your breast.

When scheduling your mammogram, you may be asked to provide your family history of breast disease. Be prepared to document who in your family has experienced breast disease, their relationship to you and their age at the time of their diagnoses. Your health care provider will use this information to assess your risk and determine a screening strategy that is right for you.

Preparing for your mammogram

You may want to schedule your mammogram for the week after your period to minimize breast pain. Taking over-the-counter pain medication one to two hours prior to your appointment can help alleviate the discomfort.

On the day of the mammogram you will be instructed to refrain from using deodorants, antiperspirants, powders, lotions or creams under your arms or on or near your breasts. These items sometimes contain metallic particles that could interfere with the quality of the images captured.

During the mammogram you'll stand in front of the X-ray device. A technician will place each breast on a platform and make the necessary adjustments to ensure the best placement possible. Your breast will be compressed. The compression helps spread out the breast tissue, making it easier to examine. It also ensures that your breast remains still so the image is not blurred. Some women find the pressure uncomfortable. If you experience too much discomfort, tell the technician. You'll be asked to hold your breath for a few seconds while the image is taken. The entire examination usually takes less than 30 minutes.

Although mammography is the most widely used method for early breast cancer detection, not all cancers are found through mammography.

Straight talk about breast density

Breast density is an important risk factor for breast cancer. Your risk of cancer is four to six times higher if you have dense breasts. Additionally, dense breasts can be challenging for traditional screening with mammography.

Dense breast tissue has less fatty tissue and more fibroglandular tissue. On a mammogram image, fatty tissue appears dark and transparent. Dense tissue, on the other hand, appears as patchy white areas. Because cancers also look white on a mammogram, having dense breast tissue makes it more difficult for radiologists to identify breast disease through standard mammography.

Dense breasts are normal and are seen in approximately 40 to 50 percent of all women who have a mammogram. Some states require, by law, that you be notified if you have dense breast tissue. Your provider may recommend supplemental screening options if you have dense breasts (see pages 205-206 for more information). The decision on whether to do supplemental screening and which test to use will take into account your cancer risk and the risks versus benefits of screening. Insurance coverage of these options varies by state and insurer.

You should never ignore a breast lump, nipple discharge or any other change in your breasts, even if your mammogram is normal.

CLINICAL BREAST EXAM A clinical breast exam (CBE) may be performed by your health care provider during a regular checkup. If used, it's typically incorporated into your annual physical beginning in your 20's and repeated every one to three years.

During the CBE, your health care provider will visually inspect your breasts while you're in a seated or standing position. He or she will be looking for changes in the shape, size or appearance of your breasts.

As estrogen levels drop with menopause, there's a reduction in the glandular tissue of the breasts and an increase in fatty tissue. Breasts will often change shape as the breast tissue becomes less elastic. You may notice that your breasts sag more, have a noticeable elongated shape or flattened appearance, or that the relative position of your nipples in relationship to your breasts changes. It's important that you share with your health care provider any visual changes to your breasts that you've noticed so that he or she can assess those changes during your exam.

Your health care provider will also carefully feel (palpate) your breasts for any lumps or abnormalities. During this part of the physical exam, you'll be lying down. Your provider will make note of any changes to the texture or appearance of the skin of your breasts or nipples. He or she may also feel under each arm to determine if you have enlarged lymph nodes.

It's important to remember that a lump does not necessarily indicate cancer. Normal breast tissue can feel lumpy, especially as breasts change in response to hormone fluctuations. Guide your health care provider to any abnormalities you may have noticed. Additionally, ask your provider to guide you to any lumps or changes in breast texture he or she identifies during your exam. This will help you become familiar with your breasts and recognize subtle changes. If a lump is found, additional evaluation may be required.

OTHER SCREENING METHODS While mammography is the best screening option for most women, additional techniques may be recommended if you are at high risk of breast cancer or have dense breasts. They include:

Breast self-awareness

Most health care providers consider breast self-examination (BSE) optional for women at average risk of breast cancer. That's because recent research has failed to show that regular breast self-exams reduce the number of breast cancer deaths. Further, other studies have shown that women who regularly perform BSE are more likely to have additional imaging tests and biopsies than women who don't perform BSE regularly.

That doesn't mean that you should not check your breasts. Breast self-awareness is still important. Breast self-awareness is a two-part process. The first requires that you become familiar with your breasts, their appearance, texture and size, and take notice when there are changes. The second requires that you know how to respond to the changes that you observe in your breasts, seeking medical attention when warranted.

Premenopausal and perimenopausal women should remember that breast tissue changes throughout the month in response to changes in your hormone levels. You may find that examining your breasts is more comfortable immediately after your period.

Breast tomosynthesis This procedure is sometimes referred to as 3-D mammography because it uses the same technology as digital mammography but takes multiple images of the entire breast to create a 3-D image. This allows radiologists to see different layers of tissue within the breast and view details within the breast tissue at different angles. Breast tomosynthesis is most often used in combination with digital mammography and may reduce the number of false-positive results from film or digital mammography alone, thereby reducing the need for additional imaging.

Ultrasound This imaging method, also called sonography, uses sound waves to create an image of tissue. Breast ultrasound is most commonly used as a diagnostic tool to further evaluate abnormalities, such as a lump, that were identified on a mammogram or through a CBE. Ultrasound can be very useful in distinguishing a benign breast condition, such as a cyst, from a more suspicious mass that would require a biopsy.

Molecular breast imaging (MBI) This procedure, also known as a nuclear medicine study, uses tiny amounts of an intravenously injected radioactive tracer that's picked up mainly by tumor cells. The tracer is injected into a vein in your arm. A special camera detects the tracer in your breasts and produces images in areas where it has accumulated abnormally. Side effects are minimal. The radiation dose is very low, and the tracer usually leaves your body within a few hours. This test is used as a screening tool and is useful for women with dense breasts.

Magnetic resonance imaging (MRI) MRI is a procedure that uses magnetic fields and radio waves, rather than radiation, to create a multi-dimensional image of the breasts. A contrast material, delivered into a vein through an IV, is used to enhance the appearance of tissues and blood vessels, which can help locate and identify tumors. Breast MRI is generally considered more sensitive than mammography and may be able to pick up some breast cancers that are not visible through mammography. It's not a perfect tool and can result in false-positive test results, leading to the need for additional imaging with ultrasound and other tests. MRI is used to screen women at high risk of breast cancer who meet certain criteria.

SCREENING CONTROVERSIES AND RISKS Breast cancer death rates have dropped 34 percent since 1990. This decline has been attributed to earlier detection through screening — specifically mammography — and more-effective treatment. You might wonder then how soon you should start screening for breast disease, and how often to repeat screening. Unfortunately, there's not a clear answer to this question.

Visual breast changes to look for

The following changes should be discussed with your health care provider.

▶ **Dimpling.** A puckering or retraction of the skin on the surface of the breast. The layer of skin on top of the breast may appear uneven and resemble the appearance of cellulite or a golf ball.

▶ **Inflammation.** Localized swelling in the breast that may appear red and sore. This swelling occurs quickly, within a day or two, and often looks like an infection of the breast. Your skin may be firm and warm to the touch. The inflammation may only affect one breast and could be accompanied by other symptoms such as a lump or changes in skin texture or appearance such as bruising or other discoloration of the skin.

▶ **Nipple retraction.** Some women are born with inverted nipples that appear indented into the breasts. New onset nipple retraction occurs when a woman whose nipples were previous raised above the surface of the breast experiences changes in the position or appearance of the nipple in relationship to the breast.

▶ **Nipple discharge.** Clear or bloody discharge either spontaneously from the nipple or by lightly squeezing the nipple doesn't necessarily predict significant disease such as cancer, but should always be evaluated.

▶ **Peau d'orange changes.** These are changes to the texture of the skin covering the breast, making the skin feel like and resemble an orange peel.

▶ **Rash on nipples.** May resemble eczema and leave the nipples looking red and scaly. Nipples may become more itchy and sensitive. Any rash on the nipple or the surrounding pigmented skin (areola) must be evaluated.

In 2009, the U.S Preventive Services Task Force (USPSTF) updated its position on breast cancer screening. It advised that women wait until age 50 to begin regular screening mammography. USPSTF also recommended that screening mammography be done every two years rather than annually. The task force cited evidence that early screening and more-frequent screening could have negative consequences that may outweigh the benefits.

Screening guidelines

The chart below provides a summary of the latest recommendations for breast cancer screening for women at average risk who have no symptoms.

Age	American Cancer Society recommendation	U.S. Preventive Services Task Force recommendation
Women in their 20s and 30s	No routine screening	No routine screening
Women ages 40 to 44	Individualized decision to begin mammogram every year	Individualized decision to begin mammogram every two years
Women ages 45 to 49	Mammogram every year	Individualized decision to begin mammogram every two years
Women ages 50 to 54	Mammogram every year	Mammogram every two years
Women ages 55 to 74	Mammogram every two years (or annually, if preferred)	Mammogram every two years
Women age 75 and older	Mammogram every two years (or annually, if preferred), as long as the individual is in good health and has a life expectancy of 10 years or longer	No recommendation

For years, many medical organizations — including the American Cancer Society (ACS), American College of Radiology and Mayo Clinic — chose not to adopt the USPSTF recommendations and continued recommending screening with annual mammography beginning at age 40. However, in 2015, the ACS updated its breast cancer screening guidelines. The new guidelines shifted the recommended starting age for annual mammography for women at average risk from 40 to 45. In addition, the ACS recommended that women age 55 and older be screened every two years instead of every year, and to continue biennial screening as long as they're in good health and are expected to live at least 10 more years. The ACS also recommended that women ages 40 to 44 and over age 55 have the option of annual screening based on their personal preferences. Finally, the ACS chose to no longer recommend clinical breast exams for women of average risk at any age.

It's important to note that these guidelines are not intended for women with breast symptoms or changes or for those at high risk of breast cancer. Mayo Clinic recommends shared decision making between women and their health care providers when considering the timing of screening.

In general, data show that women between the ages of 50 to 74 experience the greatest benefits from screening. This is because your risk of breast cancer increases as you age. Mammograms are good at identifying cancers early, before symptoms present and when treatment can be more effective and potentially less aggressive. In addition, the risks of mammography are greater for younger women. Studies have shown that women in their 40s who participate in regular screening mammograms are more likely to have false-positive results, meaning the test identifies a concern that winds up not being cancer. False-positive results lead to increased expense and anxiety for women as additional tests are ordered. Mammography is much less effective at identifying cancer in dense breast tissue than in fatty tissue. This may be a problem for younger women, who tend to have a greater amount of dense breast tissue. Mammography may also detect certain types of cancer that grow so slowly that they may never pose a threat.

Mammography is a useful screening tool. But deciding when to begin screening is a personal decision. Weigh your risk factors and discuss with your health care provider which screening methods are best for you.

Risk assessment

Many women want to understand what their chances are of developing breast cancer and if there's anything that they can do to reduce their risk.

Understanding your personal risk of developing breast cancer can help you and your health care provider make decisions about how often you should be screened, what screening methods should be used and what types of risk-reduction strategies you should consider.

Estimating breast cancer risk is difficult because researchers don't fully understand how certain risk factors affect breast health in individual women. Researchers cannot say for certain why one woman develops breast cancer and why another woman does not.

Cancer begins when there is a change (mutation) in a cell that causes the cell to grow out of control. The mutation may be inherited — passed down from a parent to a child — or it may occur spontaneously in response to aging, environmental factors or without a known cause. Many women diagnosed with cancer are often surprised since they don't have a family history of cancer. The truth is, most cancer is not hereditary. In fact, only 5 to 10 percent of breast cancers are the result of inherited genetic mutations. In addition, having a genetic mutation doesn't mean that you will develop cancer, just that you are more likely to develop cancer when combined with other factors.

COMMON RISK FACTORS There are risk factors for breast cancer that you can control and others that you cannot. Here's a look at some of them:

▶ **Sex.** Both women and men have breast tissue. However, breast cancer is 100 times more common in women than men. This is because women have more breast cells than men do and those cells are constantly exposed to higher levels of the hormone estrogen, which stimulates breast growth.

▶ **Age.** Your likelihood of having breast cancer increases as you get older.

▶ **Family history.** Having one female first-degree relative — such as a mother, sister or daughter — who has been diagnosed with breast cancer increases your own risk. The age of your first-degree relative at the time of her diagnosis is also important. In general, your risk of breast cancer increases with the number of first- and second-degree relatives who have been diagnosed with breast cancer and increases further still the younger those relatives were at the time of their diagnoses. While family history is a very significant risk factor for breast cancer, 85 percent of women with breast cancer do not have a family history of the disease.

What level of risk are you?

Women with average risk have

- No personal history of breast cancer
- No previous history of certain types of benign breast disease, including atypical hyperplasia or lobular carcinoma *in situ*
- No family history of breast cancer in a first-degree relative of either sex (parent, sibling or child) or family history of ovarian cancer in a first-degree female relative
- No previous chest radiation therapy

Women at increased or high risk have

- A personal history of breast cancer
- A past diagnosis of proliferative benign breast disease such as atypical hyperplasia or lobular carcinoma *in situ*
- Dense breast tissue
- A history of chest radiation while a child or young adult, such as the radiation used to treat lymphoma

Women at very high risk have

- Genetic testing results that indicate a BRCA1 or BRCA2 mutation or other genetic predisposition to breast cancer, or a family history of those mutations and not previously tested

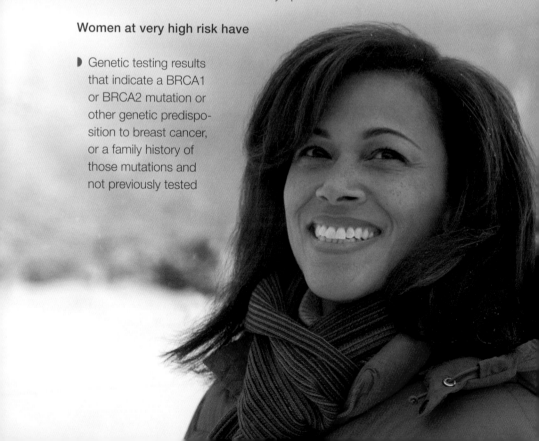

▶ **Genetic mutations.** Certain inherited changes in your genes (mutations) increase the risk of breast cancer. The most common mutations are found on two specific genes: BRCA1 and BRCA2. These mutations can be inherited from a parent of either sex. There are other gene mutations that can lead to inherited breast cancer risk, but they are much less common and don't increase your overall risk as much as a BRCA mutation.

▶ **Breast density.** Your breast cancer risk increases with your level of breast density. In fact, breast cancer risk for women with dense breast tissue is four to six times higher than for women with nondense breasts. Dense breasts also impact the effectiveness of a mammogram, as cancers may be missed on mammograms done on women with dense breasts.

▶ **Radiation therapy.** Women who, as children or young adults, were treated with chest radiation for another cancer such as lymphoma have increased risk.

▶ **Previous history of breast cancer.** If you've survived breast cancer, you are at greater risk of another breast cancer diagnosis.

▶ **Menstrual history.** The ages at which you start and end menstruation influence your risk of breast cancer. Women who began menstruating before the age of 12 or finish menstruating after the age of 55 have increased risk. The increased risk may be related to longer duration of hormone exposure through a greater number of menstrual cycles.

▶ **Race and ethnicity.** There are certain groups that are more likely to develop breast cancer or be diagnosed with more-aggressive forms of breast cancer. Black women, compared to white women, have lower rates of breast cancer, but they're more likely to be diagnosed before age 40 with cancers that are fast growing and more difficult to treat. Hispanic women also have a lower diagnosis rate than white women. BRCA1 and BRCA2 mutations are more common in women of Ashkenazi Jewish ancestry.

Risk factors that you can control are more aptly described as lifestyle factors. These will be covered in more detail later on in this chapter.

RISK MODELS Researchers have developed computer models to predict or estimate a woman's risk of breast cancer. These models are based on data collected from many women in clinical studies. Each model considers various risk factors and can help you and your health care provider make decisions about screening, testing and other options that may reduce risk and protect breast health. Here are a few of the most common models:

The Gail model The Breast Cancer Risk Assessment Tool, which is based on the Gail model, is one of the most widely used and studied tools. This model estimates the likelihood that a woman with certain risk factors will develop invasive breast cancer. Eight questions in the model capture specific risk factors including history of previous breast cancer diagnosis, current age, age at first period, age at first live birth, number of first-degree relatives (mother, sister or daughter) with breast cancer, number of previous biopsies, race, and known BRCA1 or BRCA2 genetic mutations. Critics of this model say that while it works well in its ability to predict if a group of women with similar risk factors will have an increased risk of developing breast cancer compared to the general population of women, it isn't very accurate in predicting an individual woman's risk.

The Claus model This model is similar to the Gail model but captures more details about first- and second-degree relatives' history of cancer. The Claus model is used to look at the lifetime probability as well as the 10-year probability of developing breast cancer for a woman with a documented family history of at least one female relative with breast cancer. Like the Gail model, it has its limitations — it doesn't take into account other risk factors such as the woman's age at the beginning of menstruation, biopsy history, or lifestyle factors such as pregnancy history, weight and experience with breast-feeding.

The Tyrer-Cuzick model This model provides a 10-year and lifetime estimated risk of developing breast cancer, and also estimates the likelihood that a woman carries the BRCA1 or BRCA 2 gene mutations. It takes into account risk factors such as body mass index (BMI), previous benign breast disease, age at first menstruation, pregnancy history and age at menopause, in addition to a detailed family history of breast cancer. Drawbacks are its limited accessibility.

It is important to remember that all of the breast cancer risk assessment models provide risk estimates only and are designed to support and inform your health care decisions along with other assessments such as routine screening and genetic testing.

GENETIC SCREENING You may have very mixed feelings about the idea of genetic screening. Perhaps you're wondering if genetic screening is necessary for you or maybe you worry about living with the knowledge that comes from the genetic screening results. You may be unsure about how and when to talk to your children or siblings about your decision to pursue testing or the test results. The decision to proceed with genetic screening is best made with the support of a genetic counselor who will walk you through the process, help you understand the benefits and limitations, and work with you to understand the results of your tests.

The role of a genetic counselor is to help you identify whether there is a pattern of cancer that runs through your family and to discuss the benefits and limitations of specific tests, the cost and insurance coverage information, and the people in your family who would benefit the most from being tested. He or she can then guide you through the process once you have made the decision that is best for you. Genetic counselors will never push you to undergo testing, nor will they tell you what you should or shouldn't do.

If you decide to proceed with genetic testing, the test itself is relatively simple. A blood sample will be sent to a specialized lab for analysis. Depending on the complexity of the tests ordered, your results should be available in two to four weeks. Only a small percentage of individuals will test positive for a genetic mutation. Your genetic counselor will help you understand your results and identify appropriate options for reducing your risk of breast cancer going forward.

Reducing your cancer risk

What can you do to prevent breast cancer? While we have some strategies that can reduce the risk of breast cancer, and research holds promise for developing better risk-reduction strategies, there's currently no guaranteed way to prevent the disease.

For all women, irrespective of risk factors, a change in certain lifestyle habits may lower their risk to some degree. Women at high risk of breast cancer have additional options to consider, as well.

LIFESTYLE For most of us, the power of making healthy lifestyle choices and the impact of those choices on our health isn't a mystery. We know that maintaining a healthy weight, exercising regularly, eating a low-fat diet with diverse and healthy food choices, and limiting alcohol consumption are all important to our overall health. Often, the challenge is in establishing these habits.

There are specific lifestyle choices that you can make to support better breast health and limit your risk of developing breast cancer:

What about breast pain?

Nearly all women will experience breast pain (mastalgia) at some point in their lives. Breast pain can occur in one or both breasts, and may include tenderness, aching, burning, tightness, soreness or a dull heaviness. Sometimes the pain will be focused more on the side of the breast. It's also common to experience pain in the armpit or on the front of the breast, centered around the nipple.

Pain that occurs around your menstrual cycle, lasting several days and then resolving, is called cyclic mastalgia. As your menstrual cycle becomes less regular, it may be difficult to distinguish cyclical from noncyclical breast pain. Noncyclical mastalgia is breast pain that cannot be associated with the hormone changes that accompany your menstrual cycle. Post-menopausal women are more likely to experience noncyclical breast pain. This pain may be centered more in the chest wall.

It's very rare for breast pain to signal something more concerning such as breast cancer. Talk to your health care provider about any breast pain that doesn't go away after one or two menstrual cycles, or pain that persists after menopause. There are treatment options that may help. In addition, your health care provider may want to review your current medications to see if your breast pain could be a side effect of a specific drug. Caffeine in beverages or diet may also contribute to breast pain. Even a simple issue such as an improperly fitting bra could be the culprit.

Maintain a healthy weight There's little doubt about the connection between obesity and an increased risk of breast cancer. Excess body fat leads to higher levels of estrogen, which in turn increases the risk of breast cancer. Excess body weight increases your risk of other cancers too including cancers of the kidney, colon, pancreas and uterine lining. It's always beneficial to focus on a healthy weight regardless of whether you're past menopause.

Limit alcohol Another simple lifestyle choice that you can make to reduce your risk is to limit your daily alcohol consumption. Having two or more alcoholic drinks a day can increase your risk of breast cancer by 20 percent. Simply practicing moderation in your consumption of alcohol — with a plan to eliminate or minimize alcohol to not more than one serving a day — can make a significant impact on your risk of developing breast cancer.

Choose a healthy diet Women who eat a Mediterranean diet supplemented with extra-virgin olive oil and mixed nuts may have a reduced risk of breast cancer. The Mediterranean diet focuses mostly on plant-based foods, such as fruits and vegetables, whole grains, legumes, and nuts.

Exercise regularly Aim for at least 30 minutes of exercise on most days of the week.

ASSESS HORMONE THERAPY As you learned in Chapter 10, combination hormone therapy may increase the risk of breast cancer (although by less than other risk factors such as obesity or consuming two or more alcoholic drinks a day). This doesn't mean you should avoid hormones — if you experience bothersome signs and symptoms during menopause, the increased risk may be acceptable in order to find relief. But this is why it's important to talk to your health care provider about the benefits and risks.

RISK-REDUCING MEDICATIONS If you've discovered that you're at high risk of developing breast cancer, you may want to consider this option. Chemoprevention — risk reduction using one of several medications — is best suited for women who:

▶ Have received a risk model score greater than the general population
▶ Have had a recent biopsy that identified a high-risk condition such as lobular carcinoma *in situ* or atypical hyperplasia
▶ Are at least 35 years old and have a strong family history of cancer
▶ Are positive for BRCA1 or BRCA2 mutations

However, there are often side effects to risk-reducing medications that may make the benefit not worth the risk for you. In addition, using the drug doesn't guarantee that you'll never develop breast cancer. You'll still need to keep up with regular breast screening.

Here's a look at some of the drugs used for chemoprevention:

Tamoxifen This drug is within a class of drugs called selective estrogen receptor modulators (SERMs) — drugs that change how estrogen inter-acts with breast cells by blocking estrogen from signaling cell growth in breast cells. Tamoxifen is one of the most studied SERMs used today. It's used to both treat estrogen sensitive breast cancer and reduce the risk of recurrence. Tamoxifen is frequently given as a pill that you take once a day, typically for five years. The effects of tamoxifen on cancer prevention may continue for 10 years or longer after the medication has been stopped.

Women under the age of 50 without a BRCA1 mutation will experience the greatest preventive benefits from tamoxifen. Side effects include hot flashes, blood clots and increased risk of stroke and cataracts. While tamoxifen blocks the effects of estrogen in breast tissue, it mimics the effects of estrogen on uterine tissue, slightly increasing the risk of uterine (endometrial) cancers. Antidepressants known as selective serotonin reuptake inhibitors (SSRIs) may interact with tamoxifen and impact its effectiveness. Tamoxifen can be used by both premenopausal and postmenopausal women.

Raloxifene Raloxifene (Evista) is another frequently prescribed SERM used as a risk-reducing medication for invasive breast cancer. Raloxifene doesn't increase the risk of blood clots. And because it does not simulate the effect of estrogen on the uterus, there's no added risk of endometrial cancers. While tamoxifen is more effective, raloxifene may be a better choice if you are postmenopausal and haven't had a hysterectomy. Raloxifene may also cause hot flashes.

Aromatase inhibitors (AIs) The drugs in this class — including anastrozole (Arimidex), exemestane (Aromasin) and letrozole (Femara) — reduce the amount of estrogen in your body, depriving breast cancer cells of the fuel they need to grow. They are used to treat cancer that is hormone receptor positive in women who are postmenopausal. Some women may choose to use AIs to reduce the risk of breast cancer, although the drugs aren't currently FDA-approved for this use. Although AIs aren't associated with an increased risk of blood clots or uterine cancer, they're newer medications, and not much is yet known about long-term health risks. They do increase the risk of osteoporosis, and may cause side effects such as hot flashes and vaginal dryness.

RISK-REDUCING SURGERY Women at high risk of breast cancer also have surgical options for reducing their risk. While very effective at lowering risk, they also carry significant drawbacks. The decision should be based on a thorough understanding of all options with your health care team.

Preventive mastectomy Removal of both breasts (bilateral mastectomy) is an option for women at very high risk, such as BRCA1 and BRCA2 mutation carriers or women with a strong family history that suggests a gene mutation. Women with BRCA1 or BRCA2 mutations have a lifetime risk of breast cancer of 40 to 85 percent.

Prophylactic bilateral salpingo-oophorectomy This procedure — which involves the removal of both ovaries and fallopian tubes — is generally offered to women with BRCA1 or BRCA2 mutations who are at elevated risk of ovarian cancer in addition to elevated breast cancer risk. When performed before menopause, the risk of breast cancer is also reduced.

CHAPTER THIRTEEN

Keeping your bones strong

Whether you are approaching menopause or have already transitioned beyond it, you may be concerned about your bone health. Maybe you've heard that menopause comes with significant bone loss. Or perhaps you know some women in your life who are dealing with osteoporosis, a condition that causes bones to become brittle, weak and more prone to breaks. While some bone loss is inevitable as you age, weak bones and osteoporosis are not. There are proven steps you can take to protect the health of your bones and keep them strong.

Your changing bones

Bones are living, growing tissues that are continually changing. Throughout life, old bone is broken down and removed, and new bone is formed. When you're young, your body makes new bone faster than it breaks down old bone, and your bone mass increases. Most people reach their peak bone mass by their early 30s. As you age, you lose more bone mass than is created.

Around the time of menopause, the speed at which you lose bone mass increases. A big reason for this change is a decline in estrogen, a hormone that plays an important role in building and maintaining bone. It's estimated that women lose bone mass most rapidly beginning the year or two before menopause and continuing for five to 10 years after menopause. From that point on, bone loss continues but at a slower rate.

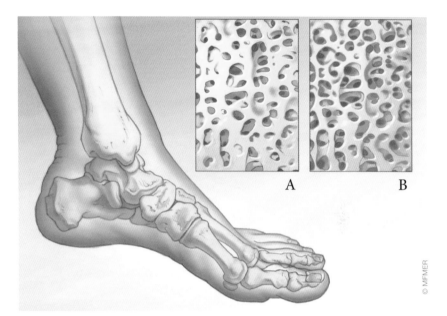

When you're young, your body makes new bone faster than it breaks down old bone, and your bone mass increases (A). As you age, you lose more bone mass than is created (B). Around the time of menopause, the speed at which you lose bone mass increases.

A loss of bone mass increases your risk of osteoporosis, which in turn increases your risk of fractures. Postmenopausal women are especially susceptible to fractures of the hip, wrist and spine. An estimated 50 percent of women over the age of 50 will break a bone due to osteoporosis.

Because osteoporosis doesn't cause obvious symptoms, it's often called a silent disease. Many women don't know they're at risk until a bone is broken. A loss in height or a stooped posture also can be a sign of osteoporosis because these changes may be due to fractures in the bones of the spine (vertebrae). Fortunately, protecting your bones and preventing osteoporosis is easier than you think — and it's never too late to start.

Evaluating your risk

You may be confident in the strength and health of your bones. Or you might be concerned about your risk of developing fractures due to bone loss. Either way, it's a good idea to take stock of your bone health in the

What affects bone health?

A number of factors affect bone health and increase the likelihood that you'll develop osteoporosis:

▶ **Gender.** Women are much more likely to develop osteoporosis than are men.

▶ **Age.** The older you get, the greater your risk of osteoporosis.

▶ **Race.** You're at greatest risk of osteoporosis if you're white or of Asian descent.

▶ **Family history.** Having a parent or sibling with osteoporosis puts you at greater risk, especially if your mother or father experienced a hip fracture.

▶ **Body frame and weight.** People who have small body frames tend to have a higher risk because they may have less bone mass to draw from as they age. A low body weight, with a body mass index (BMI) of 20 or less, also can increase your risk of developing osteoporosis.

▶ **Sedentary lifestyle.** People who are physically inactive have a higher risk of osteoporosis than do those who are more active.

▶ **Low calcium intake.** Low calcium intake contributes to lower bone mass, early bone loss and an increased risk of fractures.

early postmenopausal years. Research shows that women, especially older women, often underestimate their risk of fractures due to bone loss. In one study, more than 50 percent of patients with a moderate risk for developing fractures believed their risks were significantly lower. That number jumped to over 80 percent among patients at high risk of bone fractures.

One way to get a better sense of your bone health is to take advantage of the Fracture Risk Assessment Tool (FRAX). FRAX is a simple questionnaire that can estimate your risk of a bone fracture in the next 10 years. It was developed by the World Health Organization using data from several multithousand patient studies performed in different parts of the world.

FRAX is intended for postmenopausal women and men ages 40 to 90 who are not currently taking medications for osteoporosis. It's available free and

▶ **Tobacco and alcohol use.** Research suggests that tobacco use contributes to weak bones. Similarly, regularly having more than two alcoholic drinks a day may increase your risk of osteoporosis.

▶ **Hormone levels.** An absence of menstruation (amenorrhea) for prolonged periods before menopause can increase the risk of osteoporosis. So can entering menopause early, before the age of 45. An overactive thyroid gland or using too much thyroid hormone for an underactive thyroid can also harm bone health.

▶ **Eating disorders.** People who have anorexia or diet excessively are at risk of bone loss.

▶ **Certain medications.** Long-term use of steroid medications, such as prednisone, cortisone, prednisolone and dexamethasone, are damaging to bone. Other drugs that may increase the risk of osteoporosis include aromatase inhibitors to treat breast cancer, selective serotonin reuptake inhibitors, methotrexate, some anti-seizure medications, proton pump inhibitors and excessive amounts of aluminum-containing antacids.

Some of these risk factors are out of your control. As you'll see, though, you can lessen or even eliminate some of these risks by making small changes in your lifestyle.

online to anyone and takes into account age, sex, race, prior broken bones, family history of hip fracture, tobacco use, steroid medication use and medical conditions known to affect bone health. One way to access the tool is by going to *www.shef.ac.uk/FRAX*. Once you're there, select the "Calculation Tool" tab, choose your country of origin, and enter your personal information.

Based on your answers to the FRAX questionnaire, a computer-based algorithm will calculate your chances of having any major fracture due to osteoporosis as well as specific chances of a hip fracture in the next 10 years. Using this tool can help you and your health care provider determine when you might need further testing for osteoporosis.

FRAX can also be useful if your provider has already screened you for bone loss and determined that you have osteopenia — reduced bone density that increases your risk of developing osteoporosis. FRAX results can help you and your provider decide if and when to start preventive therapy.

Keep in mind that FRAX isn't a perfect predictor, and it can't determine whether you have osteoporosis. It's also not intended for people currently taking medication to treat osteoporosis. If you use the FRAX calculator, it's best to discuss the results with your health care provider, who can make recommendations for you based on a more thorough understanding of your particular medical history, lifestyle and circumstances.

What's the difference between osteoporosis and osteopenia?

Osteoporosis and osteopenia are both conditions relating to bone density. Having osteoporosis means that your bones are significantly weakened, increasing your risk of developing bone fractures.

If you have osteopenia, your bone density is lower than normal but not low enough to be diagnosed as osteoporosis. Having osteopenia increases your risk of osteoporosis and bone fractures, but it doesn't mean you'll end up developing the disease. The lifestyle habits described in this chapter can help prevent osteopenia from progressing to osteoporosis.

Getting your bones tested

The gold standard for assessing your risk of fracture due to bone loss is bone density testing, a fast and painless process. Bone density testing is the most accurate way to identify whether you have osteoporosis or osteopenia. When done repeatedly over time, bone density tests can also track the rate at which you're losing bone density. If you're already being treated for osteoporosis, the test can track how well your bones are responding to the treatment.

A bone density test measures the mineral content of your bones. The greater the mineral content, the denser and stronger your bones are. The most commonly used and most accurate bone density test is the dual energy X-ray absorptiometry (DXA) test. It's also known as DEXA. This noninvasive text uses low levels of X-rays. There are two types of DXA tests; a central DXA and a peripheral DXA (p-DXA). For a central DXA, you lie on a padded table as a scanner passes over your lower spine and hip. This scan is the best way to predict your risk of fractures. The p-DXA uses a smaller, portable machine to scan your wrist, fingers or heel.

Once the DXA scan measures how dense your bones are, the measurement from the scan is converted to a T-score. A T-score reflects how your bone density compares to the average peak bone density of a healthy young adult. A T-score value of 0.0 means that your bone density is equal to the average bone density of a healthy young adult. The following T-score classifications have been established by the World Health Organization:

▶ Normal — T-score above -1.0
▶ Osteopenia — T-score between -1.0 and -2.5
▶ Osteoporosis — T-score of -2.5 or lower
▶ Severe osteoporosis — T-score of -2.5 or lower with skeletal fracture

WHEN SHOULD YOU BE TESTED? It's recommended that all women have a bone density screening by age 65. Testing is also recommended if you are transitioning into menopause or are in the early years of post-menopause and have other risk factors for osteoporosis (see pages 220-221 for a list of common risk factors). If you've been taking medications that are known to cause bone loss, such as glucocorticoids, it's also recommended that you be tested.

HOW OFTEN SHOULD YOU BE TESTED? Your health care provider will recommend how often you undergo bone density testing based on your T-score and a number of other factors. If the test shows that you don't need to be treated for osteoporosis, you likely won't need to be tested again for another two to five years. If you're already taking medication to treat osteoporosis, it's recommended that you be tested again a year or two after you begin treatment to determine whether the treatment is working.

OTHER TESTS FOR BONE LOSS To get a better sense of your current bone health, your provider may suggest one or more of these additional tests:

▶ **Spinal X-rays.** Spinal X-rays can find small fractures in the spine. Spine fractures increase your risk of developing future fractures and are a strong indicator of osteoporosis. Research has shown that an adult with a fractured vertebra is five to 12 times more likely to have future fractures of the spine and two to three times more likely to break a hip. An early discovery of a fractured vertebra can lead to earlier treatment for bone loss.

Getting enough calcium in your diet

Getting calcium in the foods you eat may be easier than you think. Here are just a few examples of calcium-rich foods:

Food source	Amount of calcium in milligrams (mg)
8 ounces almond milk	451 mg
8 ounces plain, low-fat yogurt	415 mg
1 cup dry-roasted almonds	370 mg
1 cup frozen chopped collard greens, boiled	357 mg
1.5 ounces part-skim mozzarella cheese	333 mg
3-ounce can of sardines in oil	333 mg
1.5 ounces cheddar cheese	307 mg
8 ounces fat-free milk	299 mg
8 ounces soy milk	299 mg
6 ounces calcium-fortified orange juice	261 mg
½ cup whole-milk ricotta cheese	257 mg
½ cup soft tofu	253 mg
3-ounce can of salmon	181 mg
Calcium-fortified cereals	100-1,000 mg
1 cup fresh kale	100 mg

- **Computerized tomography (CT) scan.** A CT scan combines a series of X-ray images taken from different angles and uses computer processing to create cross-sectional images (slices) of the bones inside your body. CT scans might be taken of your spine, hip, forearm or lower leg. Your health care provider can use them to evaluate your bone density and identify your risk of developing bone fractures.

Preventing bone loss

Your current bone health has a lot to do with the strength of your bones in your late teens and early 20s. Adults who attained a high bone mass by their early 20s, when bones often reach their peak density, are at a lower risk of low bone density later in life.

That doesn't mean your hands are tied. While it's normal to continue losing some bone mass as you age, there are steps you can take to slow that process and prevent osteoporosis. Even if you've been diagnosed with osteoporosis, it's important to do all you can throughout your life to improve your bone health.

GOOD NUTRITION Eating a balanced diet of nutritious foods is important in maintaining an appropriate weight, which helps maintain healthy bones. In particular, the mineral calcium, along with vitamin D, is needed for healthy bones. Getting the recommended amounts of calcium and vitamin D is important throughout the rest of your life.

Calcium About 50 to 70 percent of bone tissue is made of calcium, the mineral that gives bones their hardness and strength. Getting enough calcium each day can help keep your bones strong, reduce bone loss and lower your risk of fractures. If you're a woman age 50 or younger, you need 1,000 milligrams (mg) of calcium a day. This daily amount increases to 1,200 mg when you're over the age of 50.

The preferred source of calcium is from the diet. Dairy products, dark green leafy vegetables, and calcium-fortified fruit juices and soy beverages contain good amounts of calcium. For example, an 8-ounce glass of milk or calcium-fortified soy milk contains about 300 mg of calcium. Green vegetables such as broccoli, spinach or kale provide 90 to 120 mg of calcium in a 1-cup serving when fresh or steamed.

You may need to take a calcium supplement if you're not getting enough calcium in your diet. Supplements are absorbed well and they are typically inexpensive. If you have or have had kidney stones or high blood calcium, talk to your doctor before taking calcium supplements. Taking more than 1,200 mg a day has not been shown to improve bone strength and may increase the likelihood of developing kidney stones, particularly in people who have a family history of developing them. Too much calcium taken in supplements may also be linked to heart problems. Establish a habit of taking the supplement at the same time each day, such as at bedtime or with a meal.

Vitamin D Vitamin D is an important nutrient for bone health. Vitamin D allows your body to absorb calcium by enabling it to leave your intestine and enter your bloodstream. It also works in the kidneys to help your body absorb calcium that would otherwise be excreted. In combination with calcium, vitamin D can help slow bone loss and prevent osteoporosis. The recommended daily allowance for vitamin D is 600 international units (IU) a day for adults up to age 70. When you turn 71, the recommendation increases to 800 IU a day.

Your body naturally produces vitamin D when your skin is exposed to direct sunlight. If you have light skin and you're regularly exposed to sunlight, you're likely getting some vitamin D. Keep in mind that exposing your skin to sunlight increases your risk of skin cancer. For that reason, it's a good idea to wear protective clothing and use sunscreen if you're out in the sun for more than a few minutes.

If you tend to avoid the sun or have dark skin, there are other ways to get vitamin D. Most milk is fortified with at least 100 IU of vitamin D a cup, although cheese and other dairy products usually aren't fortified. Many cereals are also fortified with vitamin D. Other good food sources include egg yolks, saltwater fish and liver. Most multivitamins also contain Vitamin D. Be aware, though, that taking too much vitamin D can be harmful. The safe upper limit for adults is 4,000 IU a day. Taking more than that may lead to high levels of calcium in the blood, which can increase your risk of kidney stones.

EXERCISE Staying physically active is another way to help prevent bone loss. Exercise has been shown to modestly increase bone density for women in midlife. It also improves posture, balance, strength and agility, all of which can prevent falls and reduce your risk of breaking a bone. What's more, exercise can help prevent disease, reduce stress, increase your energy levels and improve your overall sense of well-being.

The two types of physical activity that will most benefit your bones are weight-bearing and strength training exercises. Women who have been physically active in these ways throughout their lives generally have stronger bones than do women who have led more sedentary lives. But it's never too late to start adding exercise to your life.

Weight-bearing exercise Weight-bearing activities involve doing aerobic exercise on your feet, with your bones supporting your weight. Examples include walking, running, dancing, tennis, elliptical training machines and stair climbing. Along with strengthening your bones, these activities can provide cardiovascular benefits, which boost your heart and circulatory system health. It's worth noting that not all aerobic exercises strengthen bones. Swimming and cycling, for example, are good for your overall health but aren't considered weight-bearing exercises.

The general recommendation for adults is to get at least 150 minutes of aerobic exercise a week. That amounts to about 30 minutes on most days. Keep in mind that you don't have to do all 30 minutes at once. You can choose to exercise for shorter periods of 10 minutes three times a day.

Strength training Strength training includes the use of free weights, weight machines, resistance bands or water exercises to strengthen the muscles and bones in your arms and upper spine. Strength training can also work directly on your bones to slow mineral loss. Aim to do strengthening exercises two to three days a week. If this seems daunting, consider focusing on one area of the body each day.

When choosing among different weight-bearing and strength training exercises, know that the best exercises for your bones are the ones you enjoy doing. You'll be less likely to stick with an activity if it feels like a chore.

If you haven't exercised much and you want to get started on an exercise program, it might be a good idea to talk with your health care provider before you begin. Also consult your care provider if you've been diagnosed with osteoporosis or osteopenia, since certain activities may increase your risk of bone fractures.

OTHER LIFESTYLE CHOICES Eating well and exercising are the best ways to protect the health of your bones, but other factors also may come into play. Here are some additional steps you can take:

▶ **Avoid cigarette smoking.** Smoking speeds up bone loss and increases the chance that you'll experience a fracture. Heavy smokers are also more likely to experience early menopause. On the other hand, quitting smoking has been shown to improve bone strength.

▶ **Avoid excessive alcohol.** Research suggests that drinking moderate amounts of alcohol may strengthen bones. But consuming more than two alcoholic drinks a day may negatively affect your bone density. Being under the influence also can increase your risk of falling.

▶ **Prevent falls.** Falling doesn't affect bone density, but it does increase your risk of breaking a bone. Wear shoes that offer good support and have nonslip soles. Clear your floors of clutter and check your house for electrical cords, area rugs and slippery surfaces that might cause you to trip or fall. Keep rooms and stairwells brightly lit, and use nonslip mats in the bathtub and on shower floors.

Medications for bone loss

If you are postmenopausal and have been diagnosed with osteoporosis or have a history of broken hip bones or fractured vertebrae, your health care provider may prescribe medication to strengthen your bones in order to reduce your risk of breaking a bone. You might also receive treatment if you have osteopenia and are at a high risk of developing a bone fracture in the next 10 years. When choosing a medication, your provider will take into account your overall health, the severity of your bone loss and drugs you may be taking for other health conditions.

BISPHOSPHONATES For postmenopausal women with an increased risk of fracture, the most widely prescribed osteoporosis medications are bisphosphonates. These drugs work by slowing the rate at which your body breaks down old bone and have relatively few side effects. Bisphosphonates prescribed to strengthen bones include alendronate (Fosamax, Binosto), risedronate (Actonel, Atelvia), ibandronate (Boniva), and zoledronic acid (Reclast, Zometa). They are taken in pill form on an empty stomach daily, weekly or monthly, or intravenously once a year.

Side effects include joint or muscle pain, nausea, difficulty swallowing, heartburn, irritation of the esophagus and stomach, and ulcers in the stomach or esophagus. These are less likely to occur if the medicine is taken properly. Inflammation of the eye is an additional but rare side effect. Intravenous forms of bisphosphonates don't cause stomach upset. And it may be easier to schedule a yearly infusion than to remember to take a weekly or monthly pill, but — depending on your insurance coverage — it may be more costly to do so.

Bisphosphonates can change the structure of bone and have rarely been associated with unusual fractures of the femur. For that reason, using

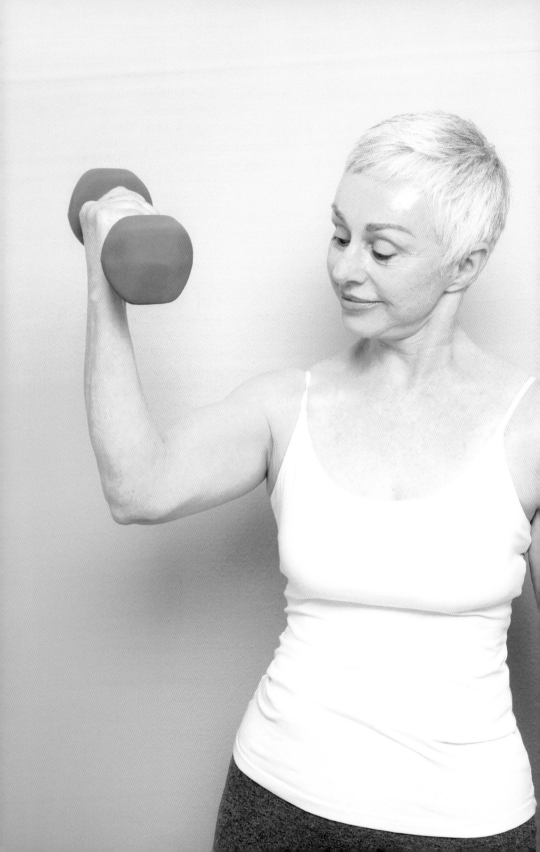

bisphosphonate therapy for more than five years has been linked to a rare problem in which the middle of the thighbone (femur) cracks or breaks.

Bisphosphonates also have the potential to affect the jawbone. Osteonecrosis of the jaw is a rare condition in which a section of jawbone dies and deteriorates, most commonly after dental procedures such as a pulled tooth, jaw surgery or dental implants. To date, it has mostly occurred in people taking high doses of an intravenous bisphosphonate to treat cancer.

RALOXIFENE Raloxifene (Evista) slows bone loss by mimicking estrogen's beneficial effects on bone density in postmenopausal women. Taking this drug may also reduce your risk of some types of breast cancer. Raloxifine comes in a daily tablet. Its side effects include hot flashes, leg cramps, blood clots, swelling and temporary flu-like symptoms.

CALCITONIN Calcitonin (Fortical, Miacalcin) is a hormone that helps to prevent bone loss and increase bone density in the spine. Because it isn't as effective as other osteoporosis medications that are available, it's generally reserved for women who aren't responding well to other treatments and are at least five years beyond menopause. It has also been shown to temporarily reduce severe pain in people who have fractured a vertebra. You can take the drug as a daily nose spray or by giving yourself daily shots under the skin or into a muscle. The nose spray can cause a runny nose, headaches, back pain and nosebleeds. Side effects of the shot are flushing of the face and hands, the need to urinate more frequently, nausea, and skin rash. The shot can also cause an allergic reaction, especially if you're allergic to salmon.

DENOSUMAB Like bisphosphonates, raloxifine and calcitonin, denosumab (Prolia) works by slowing the rate of bone loss. It's delivered with a shot under the skin every six months. The most common side effects are back and muscle pain, high levels of cholesterol in the blood, and an inflamed bladder. Denosumab may also lower the level of calcium in your blood or cause skin rashes. If you have a weakened immune system, you may also be at a higher risk of developing serious infections, especially skin infections.

TERIPARATIDE Teriparatide (Forteo) is a type of synthetic parathyroid hormone. It differs from other treatments for osteoporosis in that it helps build new bone rather than slow the loss of old bone. You take it by injecting yourself with the drug using a pre-loaded pen. Side effects include leg cramps, nausea and dizziness.

In some studies, rats receiving high doses of teriparatide developed osteosarcoma, a type of bone cancer that is very rare in humans. Although no humans to date have experienced this problem, it's not recommended that you take the drug for more than two years.

ESTROGEN Hormone therapy regimens containing estrogen can help maintain bone density, especially when started soon after menopause. Estrogen-containing hormone therapy regimens can increase your risk of blood clots, heart disease and stroke, especially when given orally. Estrogen given in combination with a progestogen is also associated with a slight increased risk of breast cancer after about five years of treatment. Estrogen is considered for treatment of low bone density or osteoporosis if you can't tolerate other medications for bone loss or if you are using it for management of bothersome menopausal symptoms. (For more information about hormone therapy, turn to Chapter 10.)

Protecting your bones for life

Although low bone density impacts the lives of many older women, you can take steps to reduce your risks and prevent or control osteoporosis. Getting enough calcium and vitamin D and taking part in regular exercise can make a real difference. If medication is needed, the good news is that a growing number of options for drug therapy are available. Research continues to offer hope for new ways to diagnose, treat and prevent bone loss.

CHAPTER FOURTEEN

Protecting your heart

With all of your questions and concerns about menopause, your heart health may not be on the top of your list. Like many people, you might think heart disease is more of a problem for men than for women. For decades, heart disease was considered a man's disease, but it's actually a problem with just as big an impact on women, if not more. In fact, heart disease is the No. 1 killer of both men and women, claiming more lives than all cancers combined. According to recent statistics, nearly 1 out of 3 women die of heart disease, and your chances of developing heart disease increase as you age, particularly once you've gone through menopause.

That may seem like sobering news, but you shouldn't let it scare you. Knowledge is power, and the information in this chapter can help you take charge of your heart health. By making healthy choices today, you can significantly reduce your risk of heart disease in the future.

Menopause and heart disease

Before menopause, women are less likely to have heart disease than are men of the same age. But once you enter menopause, your risk of heart disease increases significantly. Menopause itself doesn't cause heart disease, but declining levels of estrogen may play a role. Estrogen is thought to have a protective effect on a woman's blood vessels.

Aging also may have a significant impact on the health of your blood vessels. As you age, your arteries become less flexible. Stiff arteries are not as effective at maintaining a healthy blood flow, so your heart has to work harder to pump blood throughout your body. After menopause you're also more likely to develop conditions that increase your risk of heart disease, including high cholesterol, high blood pressure and weight gain.

Going through menopause early has an even greater effect on your chances of developing heart disease. If you've experienced menopause between the ages of 40 and 45, your risk of heart disease doubles compared with that of women your age who haven't yet gone through menopause. (More information about hormone therapy and the heart is found on page 243.)

All of this news might be unsettling, but you can do a great deal to reduce your risk of heart disease. Many of the most significant risk factors for heart disease are ones you can control. That's true at any age, regardless of when you experience menopause. Knowing about these risks — and dealing with them in a proactive way — can make all the difference.

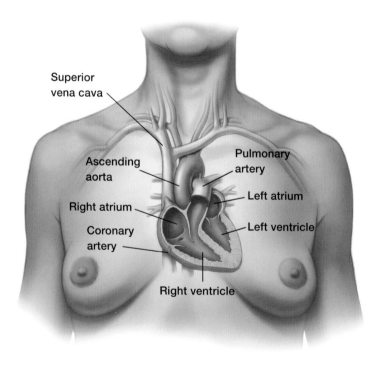

A look inside your heart

Knowing your risks

According to the American Heart Association, 90 percent of women have one or more risk factors for developing heart disease. Many of these risks factors are ones you're more likely to face in your postmenopausal years, but there's a lot you can do to reduce these risks.

HIGH CHOLESTEROL Cholesterol is a fat found in the bloodstream and in all your body's cells. Cholesterol comes from two sources. It's produced in your body, mostly in the liver, and it's found in foods that come from animals, such as meats, poultry, fish, seafood and dairy products.

Cholesterol often gets a bad rap, but it's an important part of a healthy body. Your body uses it to build cells and certain hormones. Cholesterol becomes a problem and a major risk factor for heart disease when there's too much of it in your blood. Cholesterol can build up in your arteries, increasing the risk of a blood clot forming and blocking blood flow to critical organs such as the brain (stroke) and the heart (heart attack).

Cholesterol is carried through your blood, attached to proteins. This combination of proteins and cholesterol is called a lipoprotein. You may have heard of different types of cholesterol, based on what type of cholesterol the lipoprotein carries. Here are lipoproteins commonly tested for:

▶ **Low-density lipoprotein (LDL).** This is often called "bad" cholesterol. The levels of LDL in your blood tend to increase once you reach meno-

Heart problems that are more common in women

Women are much more likely than men to have certain heart problems. The good news is that these conditions are treatable, although often more difficult to diagnose.

SMALL VESSEL DISEASE Small vessel disease is sometimes called microvascular disease or small vessel heart disease. It develops when the small arteries in your heart become narrowed so that they don't expand properly when you're active. This inability to expand is called endothelial dysfunction, and it increases your risk of heart attack. Small vessel disease is most common in perimenopausal and menopausal women. This may be due to a drop in estrogen levels combined with other risk factors for heart disease, such as high blood pressure, high cholesterol levels and diabetes.

Although it's sometimes difficult for health care providers to detect this condition, small vessel disease can be successfully treated with changes in lifestyle and medication. Typically, procedures to open the arteries are not done for this condition due to the small size of the arteries involved. Warning signs of the disease are similar to those of a heart attack. They include chest pain or discomfort; upper body discomfort in the arms, back, neck, jaw, or upper stomach; shortness of breath; nausea; and sleep problems or fatigue. If you experience these symptoms, call right away for emergency medical help.

BROKEN HEART SYNDROME Broken heart syndrome is sometimes called takotsubo cardiomyopathy, apical ballooning syndrome or stress cardiomyopathy. This acute heart condition is often brought on by stressful situations, such as the death of a loved one or even an acute illness. It involves a disruption of your heart's normal pumping function, which may be caused by your heart's reaction to a surge of stress hormones. The vast majority of people who experience this condition are menopausal women. If you experience broken heart syndrome, you may have sudden chest pain or shortness of breath and think you're having a heart attack. Indeed, it is a type of a heart attack, but not caused by a blockage in the coronary artery. These symptoms are treatable, and the reduction in heart pumping function is usually temporary, resolving completely within days or weeks. However, it may be fatal, especially in very elderly women. Medications are used to treat the weakened heart muscle until it returns to its normal function.

pause. Too much LDL cholesterol can lead to a buildup of plaque in the arteries (atherosclerosis), increasing your risk of heart attack or stroke.

▶ **High-density lipoprotein (HDL).** HDL is known as "good" cholesterol because a high level of HDL protects against heart attacks, while a low HDL level is linked to a greater risk of heart attacks. Some experts believe HDL removes excess cholesterol from arteries and carries it back to the liver to be broken down and removed from your body. Estrogen raises HDL levels, which may be why women tend to have higher levels of HDL than men do. When you reach menopause, HDL levels tend to decline. However, having high HDL doesn't mean that you're not at risk of ever having a heart attack or stroke.

▶ **Triglycerides.** Cholesterol that's produced in the liver is released into the bloodstream to supply body tissues with a type of fat called triglycerides. Triglycerides are stored in your fat cells and released for energy between

Signs and symptoms of heart disease in women

In recent years, it's been discovered that heart disease symptoms in women can sometimes differ from those in men. That knowledge has improved the diagnosis and treatment of heart disease in women. It has also empowered women to seek help sooner rather than later.

For many women, the first symptom of heart disease is a heart attack. The most common heart attack symptom in both men and women is some type of pain or discomfort in the chest. Women often describe the chest pain as a pressure, tightness or fullness. But the chest pain isn't always severe or even the most noticeable symptom. Instead, you may experience:

▶ Neck, jaw, shoulder, upper back or abdominal discomfort
▶ Shortness of breath
▶ Right arm pain
▶ Nausea or vomiting
▶ Sweating
▶ Lightheadedness or dizziness
▶ Unusual fatigue

If you experience these symptoms or think you're having a heart attack, call for emergency medical help immediately.

meals. It's the triglycerides that are measured in the lipid panel when your cholesterol is checked. Having high triglycerides results in a greater risk of heart disease in women than men.

You're more likely to have high cholesterol if it runs in your family. Being overweight, eating a diet high in saturated and trans fats, and leading a sedentary lifestyle also increase your risk. The American Heart Association recommends having your cholesterol levels checked every four to six years, starting at age 20. If you're at increased risk of developing high cholesterol, your health care provider may suggest checking earlier or testing more often.

BLOOD PRESSURE High blood pressure (hypertension) is another condition that increases your risk of developing heart disease. Hypertension is when the pressure in your blood vessels is too high. Over time, this pressure can damage your arteries, leading to an increased risk of serious conditions such as heart attack and stroke.

Blood pressure is determined by the amount of blood your heart pumps and the amount of resistance to blood flow in your arteries. The more blood your heart pumps and the narrower your arteries, the higher your blood pressure. Before menopause, your chances of having high blood pressure are lower than those of men your age. But after menopause, you're more likely to develop high blood pressure compared with your male peers, especially once you've turned 65. This can be true even if you've had normal blood pressure throughout your life. Changes in your body after menopause, including lower estrogen levels and increased body weight, contribute to higher blood pressure.

Along with your age, your chances of having high blood pressure increase if the condition runs in your family or if you're black. Your lifestyle also can play a role. For example, if you are physically inactive, eat a diet high in fats, sugars and salt, smoke or are overweight, you're more likely to develop high blood pressure.

DIABETES Diabetes also is strongly linked to heart disease, and your chances of developing it increase as you age. Having diabetes doubles your risk of having a heart attack or stroke. If you have diabetes, you're also more likely to have other risk factors that increase your risk of heart disease, such as high blood pressure, high cholesterol and obesity.

The term *diabetes* refers to a group of diseases that affect the way your body uses blood sugar, also called glucose. The most common forms of

Know your blood pressure numbers

You can have hypertension for years without any symptoms. That's why it's so important to have your blood pressure checked regularly. If you discover you have high blood pressure, you can work with your health care provider to control it.

A blood pressure reading contains a top number and a bottom number. The top number is the systolic measurement. Your systolic reading tells you the pressure in your arteries during a heartbeat, when your heart is pushing blood through your arteries. The bottom number is the diastolic measurement. This number represents the pressure in your arteries when your heart is at rest between heartbeats. Your systolic number will be higher than your diastolic number.

Blood pressure readings are broken down into several categories:

Your category	Systolic (mm Hg) (top number)	Diastolic (mm Hg) (bottom number)
Normal	Less than 120	Less than 80
Prehypertension	120 to 139	or 80 to 89
Hypertension Stage 1 Stage 2	140 to 159 160 or higher	or 90 to 99 or 100 or higher
Hypertensive crisis (seek emergency care immediately)	Higher than 180	Higher than 110

Based on Chobanian AV, et al. Seventh report of the Joint National Committee on Prevention, Detection, Evaluation, and Treatment of High Blood Pressure. *Hypertension.* 2003;42:1206.

Keep in mind that one high reading isn't enough for your provider to determine that you have high blood pressure. High blood pressure is diagnosed when you've had several high readings over a period of time. There's no cure for high blood pressure, but the healthy lifestyle habits discussed later in this chapter can help you prevent or manage the condition. Your health care provider may also prescribe medication to lower your blood pressure if you have stage 1 or stage 2 hypertension. If you're concerned about your blood pressure, make an appointment to discuss it with your provider.

diabetes are type 1 and type 2. Type 1 diabetes most often develops in children and young adults. Type 2 diabetes develops more commonly in midlife and beyond, and is associated with increased body weight. If you have diabetes, it means your body can't produce enough insulin or it can't use insulin properly. When that happens, the glucose in your bloodstream is unable to enter your cells, which results in a potentially dangerous buildup of glucose in your bloodstream.

Because symptoms of type 2 diabetes can be mild or nonexistent, it's common to be unaware that you have the condition. The American Diabetes Association recommends being regularly screened for diabetes if you are 45 or older. If the results of your test are normal, you should get retested every three years. If the test indicates that your blood sugar levels are higher than normal, your doctor will likely want to test you on a yearly basis.

Your risk of developing type 2 diabetes increases if the disease runs in your family. Being overweight or obese, not getting enough exercise, and eating an unhealthy diet also increase your chances of diabetes. Managing these risks with a healthy lifestyle will not only help you prevent or manage diabetes but also lower your risk of heart disease.

YOUR FAMILY HISTORY You've probably noticed that many of the conditions that increase your risk of heart disease run in families. The same is true for heart disease itself, especially if a close relative developed heart disease at an early age.

As you reach menopause, it's a good idea to gather information about your family's medical history and share it with your health care provider. Make sure your provider knows about parents, siblings and grandparents who've had heart disease and other conditions that increase your own risk, including high cholesterol, high blood pressure and diabetes. If heart disease does run in your family, it's more important than ever to protect your heart health by making good choices and controlling the risk factors that you can.

Heart protection strategies

You may not be able to change your age or your family history, but there's a lot you can do to prevent heart disease. Taking charge of your heart health now will allow you to enjoy a rich and satisfying life for years to come.

ASPIRIN AND HEART DISEASE You may have heard that an aspirin a day keeps heart disease at bay. That's because aspirin can reduce your chances of developing a blood clot in your arteries. If your arteries are narrowed, a blood clot can prevent blood flow to your heart or brain and cause a heart attack or stroke. But aspirin can have serious side effects, including internal bleeding.

Diagnosing heart disease in women

For decades, the stress test — in particular the exercise stress test — has been the gold standard for noninvasive testing of heart disease. The test usually involves walking on a treadmill or riding a stationary bike while your heart rate, heart rhythm and blood pressure are monitored.

The stress test can be an effective way to identify heart disease in both men and women, but some women may also benefit from additional testing. That's because women are more likely than men to develop small vessel disease, which is not as easily identified using a stress test. Unlike atherosclerosis, which blocks blood flow to the heart and major arteries, small vessel disease results from damage to small arteries or the inner lining of the main arteries leading to the heart. Research has shown that this condition can increase the risk of serious heart disease.

For this reason, imaging techniques — such as magnetic resonance imaging (MRI), positron emission tomography (PET), echocardiography or specialized vascular tests to evaluate the health of the lining of the blood vessels (endothelial testing) — may be recommended in addition to a stress test for women with symptoms of heart disease.

A major study called the Women's Health Study (WHS), which began in 1993 and ended in 2004, looked at the use of low-dose aspirin for the prevention of heart disease in women. The WHS indicated that the benefits may not outweigh the risks for women under the age of 65 who have no history of heart disease. Although a regular low dose of aspirin did reduce the risk of stroke in that category of women, it didn't significantly reduce the risk of heart attack. Based on these findings, the North American Menopause Society and the American Heart Association do not recommend taking a daily dose of aspirin to prevent heart attack if you're a woman under 65 without existing heart disease.

Guidelines are varied among other organizations and are evolving as more research is done. The bottom line is that you should have a discussion with your health care provider before taking a daily dose of aspirin. Based on your medical history and any medications you may be taking, he or she will be able to determine whether using aspirin to prevent heart disease is a good option for you. Of course, if you have already had a heart attack, a daily baby aspirin is recommended for life, unless you have significant reasons for not doing so.

STATINS If you have high cholesterol, it's smart to be proactive when it comes to heart disease. Changes in your diet and exercise routine may be enough to get your cholesterol levels under control. If not, your health care provider may suggest that you take a statin.

Statins are drugs that work by blocking a substance your body needs to make cholesterol. Statins may also help your body reabsorb cholesterol that has built up in plaques on your artery walls, preventing further blockage in your blood vessels and lowering your risk of heart attacks. Statins include medications such as atorvastatin (Lipitor), fluvastatin (Lescol), lovastatin (Altropev), pitavastatin (Livalo), pravastatin (Pravachol), rosuvastatin (Crestor) and simvastatin (Zocor). Lower cost generic versions of many statin medications are available.

Statins and women To date, most studies have focused on the ability of statins to help prevent heart disease in men. It's not as clear whether statins produce a similar benefit for women. Recent research has raised the possibility that statins may not lower women's risk of developing heart disease, although more research is needed. However, it has been clearly shown that in women who've had a heart attack, statins prevent recurrent heart attack and prolong survival just as well as in men, if not better.

In the past, risk assessment tools didn't factor sex differences into the equation. However, current guidelines do consider that women's risk may differ from men's. The latest risk calculator, developed from guidelines by the American College of Cardiology (ACC) and American Heart Association (AHA), helps to predict your 10-year and lifetime risks of developing heart disease by taking into account several risk factors, such as blood pressure, cholesterol levels, and whether you smoke. A high 10-year risk score is one factor health care providers use to decide whether to prescribe a statin.

Current recommendations for taking statins Regardless of your sex, you should try to keep your total cholesterol level below 200 milligrams per deciliter (mg/dL) — or 5.2 millimoles per liter (mmol/L), as measured in some countries. LDL cholesterol should be below 100 mg/dL (2.6 mmol/L).

Because statins can help to reduce LDL cholesterol, they are recommended for certain groups of people. The ACC/AHA guidelines focus on four main groups who may be helped by statins:

- **If you already have heart disease.** If you've had a heart attack, stroke caused by blockages in a blood vessel, ministroke (transient ischemic attack), peripheral artery disease, or prior surgery to open or replace coronary arteries, a statin is recommended.

- **If you have very high LDL cholesterol.** If your LDL cholesterol reading is 190 mg/dL or higher, statins are recommended.

- **If you have diabetes.** If you have diabetes and an LDL reading between 70 and 189 mg/dL, especially if you have signs of vascular disease, you may want to consider taking statins.

- **If you have a higher 10-year risk of heart attack.** If you have an LDL reading above 100 mg/dL and your 10-year risk of a heart attack is 7.5 percent or higher, your health care provider may prescribe a statin.

Side effects of statins The most common side effect is mild muscle pain. Very rarely, statins can cause rhabdomyolysis, a serious condition that can lead to severe muscle pain or damage to your kidneys. Rhabdomyolysis can develop when you take statins in combination with certain drugs or if you take a high dose of statins. Statins also are associated with a slightly increased risk of diabetes, liver damage and cognitive problems such as memory loss, forgetfulness or confusion.

If you are concerned about your cholesterol levels, talk to your provider about your total risk of heart disease and discuss how your sex and lifestyle play a role in your decision about taking medication for high cholesterol.

A heart-healthy lifestyle

So far the focus of this chapter has been on medical conditions that can affect your heart health. But your lifestyle also can have a huge impact on your chances of developing heart disease. Believe it or not, about 80 percent of cardiovascular diseases can be prevented through a combination of healthy lifestyle habits. These habits include not smoking, eating a healthy diet, exercising, and maintaining a healthy weight. Many of these habits can

Hormone therapy and prevention of heart disease

Hormone therapy isn't recommended for prevention of heart disease. And if you've already developed heart disease, hormone therapy isn't right for you. But recent studies have indicated that using menopausal hormone therapy early in your menopausal years for treatment of menopausal symptoms may reduce your chances of developing heart disease. As discussed in Chapter 10, this evolving idea is called the "timing hypothesis," and it suggests that taking estrogen therapy within 10 years of menopause and before age 60 may reduce your risk of heart disease. On the other hand, taking estrogen after age 60, when some atherosclerosis is likely already present, is believed to have a harmful effect.

also prevent conditions that increase your risk of heart disease, including diabetes, high cholesterol and high blood pressure. By leading a healthy lifestyle, you'll be improving your overall health, longevity and well-being.

AVOID TOBACCO Smoking or using tobacco of any kind is one of the most significant risk factors for developing heart disease, particularly in women. Chemicals in tobacco can damage your heart and blood vessels. Using tobacco may also increase your risk of blood clots and lower your levels of HDL (the "good") cholesterol. Carbon monoxide in cigarette smoke replaces some of the oxygen in your blood. This increases your blood pressure and heart rate by forcing your heart to work harder to supply enough oxygen.

When it comes to heart disease prevention, no amount of smoking is safe. But, the more you smoke, the greater your risk. Even so-called "social smoking" — smoking only while at a bar or restaurant with friends — is dangerous and increases the risk of heart disease. So does exposure to secondhand smoke.

The good news is quitting smoking can rapidly reduce your risk. And it's never too late to quit. Women who quit smoking between the ages of 45 and 54 gain an average of six years of life compared with women who continue to smoke. Quitting smoking can also lower your risks of other diseases linked to tobacco use, such as lung cancer.

Quitting strategies If you smoke, quitting may seem like an impossible mountain to climb. You'll improve your chances of success if you get the right support. That support can come from family, friends, your health care provider, a counselor, a support group or a telephone quit line. Support can also come from using a medication for smoking cessation. Seeking out smoke-free restaurants, bars and workplaces also can make a big difference. The more committed you are to sticking with a plan, the more likely you'll be able to kick the habit.

EAT A HEART-HEALTHY DIET One of the best things you can do to protect your heart is to eat a healthy diet. Depending on your eating habits, that may mean fine-tuning your diet or making more significant changes. Taking on a new eating plan may seem daunting, but it's well worth the effort. A healthy diet can help you prevent not only heart disease but factors linked to heart disease risk, such as diabetes, high cholesterol and weight gain.

Eating well isn't just about how many calories you consume. Heart-healthy diets such as Dietary Approaches to Stop Hypertension (DASH), the Mediterranean Diet and the Mayo Clinic Diet focus on enjoying a variety of foods that meet your body's needs. Following are some tips to consider when it comes to eating for your heart health.

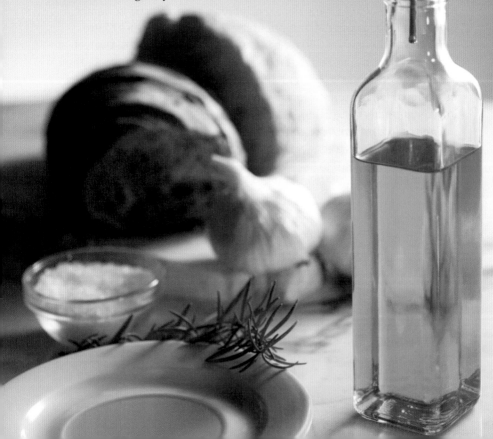

Eat more vegetables and fruits Vegetables and fruits are good sources of vitamins and minerals. Vegetables and fruits are also low in calories, rich in dietary fiber and contain substances found in plants that may help prevent cardiovascular disease. Eating more fruits and vegetables may help you eat less high-fat foods, such as meat, cheese and snack foods.

Choose whole grains Whole grains are good sources of fiber and other nutrients that play a role in regulating blood pressure and heart health. You can increase the amount of whole grains in your diet by making simple substitutions for refined grain products. Or be adventuresome and try a new whole grain, such as farro, quinoa or barley.

Limit unhealthy fats Limiting how much saturated fat you eat and avoiding trans fat in processed foods is an important step to reduce your blood cholesterol and lower your risk of heart disease. The best way to reduce saturated fat in your diet is to limit the amount of butter and other solid fats you add to food. You can also reduce the amount of saturated fat in your diet by choosing lean meats with less than 10 percent fat.

The Food and Drug Association (FDA) has recently determined that artificial trans fats are generally not safe in any amount. Trans fats have been shown to raise LDL cholesterol, increasing the risk of heart disease. The main source of artificial trans fat is partially hydrogenated oils, which are currently added to some processed foods. The FDA is requiring the food industry to phase out trans fat from most of its products by 2018.

When you do use fats, choose monounsaturated fats, such as olive oil or canola oil. Polyunsaturated fats, found in certain fish, avocados, nuts and seeds, also are good choices for a heart-healthy diet. When used in place of saturated fat, monounsaturated and polyunsaturated fats may help lower your total cholesterol.

Choose low-fat protein sources Lean meat, poultry, fish, low-fat dairy products, eggs and legumes are some of your best sources of protein. But be careful to choose lower fat options, such as skim milk rather than whole milk and skinless chicken breasts rather than fried chicken with the skin on. Fish is another good alternative to high-fat meats. And certain types of fatty fish are rich in omega-3 fatty acids, which can lower triglycerides in your blood.

Avoid excess salt Sodium is an essential mineral that your body needs to perform a variety of functions. The amount of sodium most adults need is very low (less than 500 mg daily) compared with the average intake in the U.S. (over 3,200 mg daily). Lowering how much salt you consume in the foods you eat can lower your blood pressure and reduce your risk of heart disease, while consuming too much salt can raise your blood pressure. The

American Heart Association recommends consuming less than 1,500 mg of sodium a day, but even reducing your sodium intake to 2,400 mg a day can have a positive effect on your blood pressure and heart health.

Stay away from sugary drinks and foods Too much sugar in your diet can increase your likelihood of developing heart disease. The American Heart Association recommends that women consume no more than 6 teaspoons or 100 calories of sugar a day. A can of soda contains 8.75 teaspoons or 140 calories of sugar. Drinking fewer sweetened beverages — or cutting them out altogether — is a great way to reduce the amount of sugar you consume. Also beware of foods packed with added sugar, such as bakery goods, breakfast cereal, candy and some yeast breads.

GET MOVING When it comes to your heart, healthy eating and exercise go hand in hand. While being inactive can increase your risk of heart disease as much as smoking can, physical activity not only reduces your risk but also can help you maintain a healthy weight and prevent high blood pressure, high cholesterol and diabetes. Exercising regularly will also strengthen your muscles and bones, raise your energy levels, and boost your self-confidence.

The American Heart Association recommends you get at least 150 minutes of moderate exercise, 75 minutes of vigorous exercise or a combination of both each week. Aim for at least 30 minutes of aerobic activity most days of the week. Shorter bursts of three 10-minute exercise sessions throughout the day can offer the same health benefits.

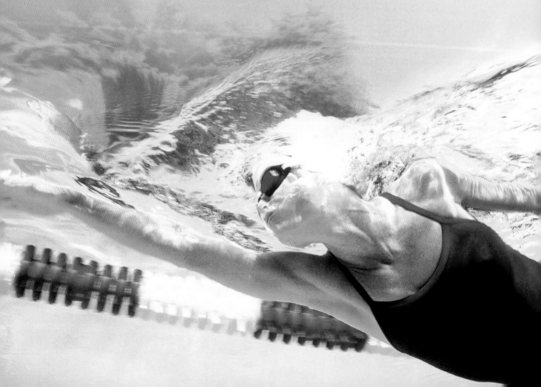

Running, swimming, bicycling and active sports such as tennis are all forms of heart-healthy aerobic activity. So are daily activities such as gardening, housekeeping, taking the stairs and walking the dog. You don't have to exercise strenuously to achieve benefits, but you can see bigger benefits by increasing the intensity, duration and frequency of your workouts. The most important thing is to avoid being inactive, so choose the activities that are most enjoyable to you.

If you haven't been exercising much, take things slowly at first. For example, start by walking for five to 10 minutes most days and gradually work your way up to 30 or more. If you have any concerns about starting a new exercise program, talk with your health care provider.

MAINTAIN A HEALTHY WEIGHT Maintaining a healthy weight is an important part of reducing your chances of developing heart disease. But as you get older, you may be noticing changes in your weight and body shape. The hormonal changes of menopause might make you more likely to gain weight around your abdomen than around your hips and thighs. Muscle mass also tends to diminish with age, while fat increases.

Even a small weight loss can be beneficial. A good goal if you're overweight is to aim to lose 5 to 10 percent of your body weight over a period of six months. For example, if you weigh 150 pounds, that's just 7 to 15 pounds. Reducing your weight by that little can help decrease your blood pressure, lower your cholesterol level and reduce your risk of diabetes. Even a lasting weight loss of 3 to 5 percent can have a positive impact on your heart health.

See Chapter 9 for specific strategies on maintaining a healthy weight in menopause and beyond.

A healthy heart for life

Now is a good time to change many of your risk factors for heart disease. Seek out the support of friends and family members who might also benefit from taking on healthier habits. Reward yourself for accomplishments, and don't be discouraged by bumps in the road. By sticking with these healthy habits, you'll be going a long way toward protecting your heart.

CHAPTER FIFTEEN

Your brain and menopause

Ask any group of women who are going through menopause whether the transition has affected their brains and the answer is likely to be an emphatic yes. Some complain of the inability to remember familiar names or common words, others of a lack of focus or concentration, and still others of forgetting where they put things — now where did those keys go again?

It's been shown that estrogen does indeed have an influence on key aspects of brain processing and metabolism. Multiple studies have been launched in an attempt to tease out the link between the hormonal fluctuations of menopause and the cognitive symptoms that commonly occur during this period. Even so, the exact relationship between the two remains unclear.

Part of the difficulty in defining the association is that menopause isn't just an isolated event. It occurs in the broader context of aging and the multiple changes that brings. Many of the physical symptoms that are common during menopause — irregular periods, hot flashes, mood swings and disrupted sleep — can have an effect on your ability to think and remember, as well. As a result, it appears that there are multiple factors at play.

Although there's still much to be discovered, this chapter will try to help you understand what's going on with your brain at this stage in your life. It will also delve into what you can do to protect that most valuable of assets — your mind.

Changes that occur with aging

Most likely, you already know that all of your egg cells were formed in your ovaries before you were even born. In a similar fashion, you were born with billions of brain nerve cells (neurons) already in place. What's more, you keep these neurons for life. Their number declines throughout life but they are capable of living for up to 100 years or longer. Amazing, right?

But neurons don't just sit there. They're abuzz with signals and messages (electric impulses) to each other, lighting up paths of communication across the brain that make today's complex transmission of wireless data look like child's play. Each neuron is designed to collect and process messages, and then relay the information to other neurons. Neuronal communication regulates actions you consciously think about, such as writing an email or talking with a friend, along with actions you don't think about, such as breathing, experiencing pain or blinking dust from your eye.

Collectively, your neurons are also a repository for instincts, memories, intellectual analyses and creative thoughts. Together, they organize and shape your emotions and guide your actions and reactions.

To stay healthy, neurons are constantly maintaining and repairing themselves. As you age, however, some of these maintenance and repair processes may start to malfunction or get out of sync. Also, trauma or disease can irreparably damage neurons.

After about the fifth or sixth decade of life, the normal brain undergoes changes that include:

▶ A loss of neurons, especially in certain areas of the brain such as the prefrontal cortex, an area at the front of the brain, and the hippocampus, a small portion found deep inside toward the center of the brain. Both of these areas are important to cognitive skills such as learning, remembering, planning and decision-making. Losing neurons means the volume of your brain shrinks (atrophies) slightly.

▶ Disruption of communication between neurons due to loss or damage.

▶ Diminished coordination between brain regions.

▶ Reduced blood flow in the brain due to narrower arteries and fewer new blood vessels.

▶ Accumulation of debris inside and around neurons.

- Increased damage from free radicals, molecules that are unstable and hyperreactive.

- Increased inflammation.

For most women, changes such as these mean becoming a little more forgetful — experiencing momentary lapses often brought on by inattention or distraction. It may be a bit harder to recall information "on the spot," for example, such as rattling off the date of a best friend's birthday or the title of a book you finished recently. And distant memories that you don't call upon often may fade even further.

You might catch yourself being more absent-minded. You become so preoccupied with one thought that you overlook everything else. Or you're doing too many things at once and forget some of them.

In addition to memory, other cognitive functions become vulnerable, such as your brain's processing speed. Your brain may require more time to solve complex problems or assess visually challenging input, compared with people in their 30s and 40s.

Your brain may also need more time to make sense of new or unfamiliar information, or you might need additional details or instruction to master a new skill.

This doesn't mean that you're not as smart as you once were or that you can no longer think for yourself. It just means you might take a little longer to figure out an answer or grasp concepts that are new to you. In fact, when given adequate time, older adults deliver solutions to problems that are just as accurate and effective as those of younger adults.

On the other hand, many important cognitive functions are hardly affected at all by the normal aging process. Generally, your ability to focus, concentrate and create aren't diminished by time. Correctly choosing your words and accessing a rich vocabulary actually improve over the years.

And don't forget the benefits that age can bring, such as wisdom and experience. In your 50s and 60s and beyond, you have much more knowledge and insight to draw upon than in previous decades.

Hormones and the brain

You're probably aware by now how influential estrogen can be. It affects many more organs and systems in your body than just your ovaries. In fact, it plays an important role in your brain health, as well.

When is forgetfulness a problem?

Occasional forgetfulness is typical of normal aging. So don't stress out too much about forgetting an appointment or misplacing a set of keys. On the other hand, forgetfulness caused by disease is new and becomes progressively worse. Early signs of cognitive impairment are often noticed by others and may include:

▶ Asking the same questions repeatedly without remembering the answer

▶ Stopping in the midst of a conversation without remembering what the discussion was about

▶ Mixing words up — saying "bed" instead of "table," for example

▶ Taking longer to complete familiar tasks, such as putting on makeup or brushing teeth

▶ Placing items in inappropriate places, such as putting the mail in the freezer

▶ Getting lost while walking or driving in familiar places

▶ Making rash decisions, such as about personal safety or money

▶ Undergoing sudden changes in mood or behavior for no apparent reason

▶ Experiencing increasing difficulty following directions

Biologic studies have pinpointed cells throughout the brain that contain estrogen receptors. Circulating estrogen binds to these special molecules that function as a gateway for estrogen to exert its influence on targeted brain cells. Basic science suggests that estrogen may have protective effects on neurons and cognitive function by:

▶ Increasing the production of acetylcholine, a chemical that neurons within the cholinergic system use to communicate with each other (neurotransmitter). The cholinergic system plays a big role in the regulation of learning and memory.

- Enhancing the glutamate neurotransmitter system, a communication route involved in long-term potentiation — how you learn new things.

- Regulating genes that influence how neurons survive, differentiate, regenerate and adapt.

- Buffering neurons from overstimulation by neurotransmitters and protecting them from harmful free radicals.

Studies of progesterone, the female hormone that has the job of counterbalancing the effects of estrogen, are fewer, but they also indicate a protective effect by progesterone on neurons.

WOMEN AND COGNITIVE DECLINE Alzheimer's disease is a progressive degeneration of the brain that involves an overwhelming loss of neurons and the connections between them. It's one of the most common illnesses of old age, and one of the most devastating.

Yet despite the protective nature of female hormones toward the brain, Alzheimer's affects many more women than men. According to the Alzheimer's Association, women make up two-thirds of American seniors living with Alzheimer's. In addition, at age 65, women have more than a 1 in 6 chance of developing Alzheimer's over the remainder of their lives, compared to men who have a 1 in 11 chance.

Why is this? One obvious reason is that women generally live longer than men, which increases their overall chances of developing Alzheimer's. But there are likely other sex differences at play, too, and scientists are only beginning to uncover what some of these might be.

Interestingly, mild cognitive impairment (MCI), a stage that often precedes Alzheimer's disease, is more prevalent in men than women. But women with MCI appear to decline at a faster rate than men, descending more abruptly into dementia. It's possible that men may experience cognitive decline earlier in life but at a more gradual pace, whereas women may rapidly proceed from normal cognition to dementia at a later age.

Estrogen plays a role, but exactly how is uncertain. It's tempting to draw a neat line between estrogen decline during the menopausal transition and increased risk of cognitive impairment. In animal studies, for example, abrupt withdrawal of estrogen results in increased cellular stress and faulty memory. On the flip side, clinical trials of younger women who take estrogen after a hysterectomy show improved verbal memory.

It would seem to make sense that replacing hormones when they're low — such as what occurs around menopause and after — would improve cognitive function and even help prevent dementia. But as discussed later in this chapter, evidence from clinical trials so far hasn't been very straightforward, and in some instances, hormone therapy has had harmful effects.

As with most diseases, Alzheimer's most likely results from a complex interplay between genetics, environment and other individual characteristics including sex, metabolism and lifestyle choices. Investigators are working to tease out what these various factors may be, as well as how the choices we make may affect the outcome.

An example of this interplay can be found in a study that focused on the links between telomeres, APOE e4 status, menopause and hormone therapy.

Telomeres are the protective endcaps on every chromosome. They're often likened to the plastic ends on a shoelace that help keep the shoelace from unraveling. In the same way, telomeres keep the DNA within a chromosome from unraveling or becoming damaged. Telomere length is often used as a measure of cellular aging. Longer telomeres are associated with greater health and longer life spans. Although women and men have similar telomere length at birth, by adulthood women generally have longer telomeres, possibly due to the beneficial effects of circulating estrogen. APOE e4 is a genetic variant that increases the risk of Alzheimer's disease.

The researchers theorized that the healthy middle-aged women participating in their study who had the APOE e4 genetic variant would display shorter telomeres at the end of a two-year period than women who didn't have this variant. They also speculated that hormone therapy, initiated at the start of the menopausal transition, would protect against telomere shortening.

Study results showed that the odds of telomere shortening over the two-year period were more than six times greater in APOE e4 carriers compared to noncarriers. In other words, cells appeared to age a lot faster in women with the APOE e4 variant.

Hormone therapy was a game changer for the APOE e4 carriers, however. APOE e4 carriers who were on hormone therapy showed little to no decline in telomere length. But for noncarriers, hormone therapy had little protective effect on cell aging. In fact, noncarriers who went off of hormone therapy experienced increased telomere length.

Results such as these need to be explored and validated by additional research. But they suggest that disease — and the medicine needed to effectively treat it — is much more individualized than previously thought.

HORMONE THERAPY AND THE BRAIN In the early 2000s, investigators published results based on several large, long-term, rigorous clinical trials on women's health. One of the largest was a clinical trial known as the Women's Health Initiative (WHI). An offshoot of this study, the Women's Health Initiative Memory Study (WHIMS) followed over 4,500 women between the ages of 65 and 79 for about four years to see what effects hormone therapy might have on cognitive health, the general assumption being one of benefit. On the contrary, however, the WHIMS trial found that use of hormone therapy in older women didn't improve cognition at all and that in fact, it was actually harmful for memory in some women.

Another offshoot study of the Women's Health Initiative, the WHI Study of Cognitive Aging (WHISCA), enrolling women 66 years and older, found neither benefit nor persistent harm on cognitive health in older women using hormone therapy.

Other, smaller studies have found similar results. The Heart and Estrogen-Progestin Replacement Study (HERS), which looked into the long-term effects of hormone therapy on cognition and heart health, found that among older postmenopausal women, hormone therapy for four years didn't result in any improvement on cognitive tests.

The publication of this data swung opinion against using hormone therapy for preventing cognitive decline, and other conditions as well, since hormone therapy was also shown to increase the risk of diseases such as stroke and breast cancer.

However, this may not be the end of the story. As mentioned in Chapter 10, women's health researchers are still sorting through the implications of these studies. A number of factors highlight the need for further investigation. For example, the increased risk of stroke was observed primarily in older women who were using oral estrogen. In addition, the risk of breast cancer was increased only in the group that took estrogen plus progestin. Breast cancer risk actually decreased in women who took estrogen alone. Caveats such as these suggest support for speculations that timing, dose, route of administration and the specific hormone therapy regimen used may play an important role in the balance of benefits and risks.

Based on current knowledge, the risks of hormone therapy use in healthy women ages 50 to 59 remain very low. On the other hand, greater risks are associated with starting hormone therapy in your 60s or 70s.

ALL IN THE DETAILS? A lot of current research revolves around the idea that there's a critical window in which hormone therapy can have positive effects. Observational studies suggest that hormone therapy used in women who are closer to the menopausal transition decreases the risk of Alzheimer's disease, whereas hormone therapy used in later years — especially a combined estrogen and progestin formulation — increases the risk.

Additionally, recent brain imaging studies of women who use hormone therapy early on in menopause reveal enhanced function of the hippocampus and prefrontal cortex, areas of the brain important for memory and thinking.

Other recent studies have yielded more-neutral results. The Kronos Early Estrogen Prevention Study (KEEPS) is a large clinical trial involving approximately 700 women who enrolled within three years of their final menstrual period — a substantially younger group than the preceding WHIMS and other studies.

An offshoot of the study, KEEPS Cognitive and Affective Study (KEEPS-Cog), evaluated the cognitive effects of hormone therapy in these women over a period of four years. Preliminary results showed that hormone therapy wasn't harmful to learning or memory but neither was it helpful. However, it did improve symptoms such as depression, tension and anxiety. Long-term follow-up of these women will hopefully yield additional clues as to the relationship between menopause, hormone therapy and cognition.

Another study, the Early Versus Late Intervention Trial With Estradiol (ELITE), is also looking into whether hormone therapy use early in menopause is more beneficial than later use.

Keeping your brain healthy

Setting aside the complexities of hormone therapy and its effects on cognition, rest assured that menopause is certainly no harbinger of mental decline. Results from long-term observational studies of women going through menopause are generally encouraging. For example, it may be comforting to know that while the natural progression toward menopause may indeed have a small yet noticeable impact on your cognitive function — provoking some of the thinking and memory difficulties you may be experiencing — such changes are not enough to make you score poorly on a memory assessment test. In addition, these menopause-related difficulties most likely are temporary and have little long-term effect on your brain health.

Scientists are just beginning to uncover factors that may help people protect their minds into their later years. One thing that's becoming increasingly clear is that changes to the brain begin much earlier than once believed and can eventually accumulate enough damage to cause severe loss of memory and thinking skills. What this also means, however, is that there most likely are measures you can take in midlife to preserve and enrich your brain health.

Three factors have emerged so far as legitimate steps you can take to preserve brain health:

PROTECT YOUR HEART Mounting evidence indicates that what's good for your heart is good for your brain, too. As one of the largest and busiest

Memory boosters

Habit-based (procedural) memory is used to store skills developed by repetition and practice — like riding a bike. It stays with you all your life.

You can capitalize on procedural memory skills to sharpen everyday memory skills and speed up information processing. This in turn allows you to take full advantage of other invaluable skills, such as insight and experience, which can only be acquired over time. Here's how:

KEEP A CALENDAR Like most women these days, you're probably bombarded with lots of information coming from all directions — names, numbers, passwords, to-do lists. Trying to track too many tedious details can actually make you more prone to memory lapses.

Instead, create an effective calendar and organization system to help you keep extraneous information readily available and yet free up brain space for more important tasks. There are a variety of tools that can help you organize and remember appointments and tasks — from paper calendars to notebooks to apps. The most important thing is to pick one and use it regularly, to the point where it becomes a habit — this is how procedural memory can make up for faulty recent memory.

It also helps to categorize the information you're trying to remember. Instead of one big long list, create separate sections for scheduled events, tasks that need to get done, and static information such as phone numbers, addresses and other contact information.

ORGANIZE THE CLUTTER Keeping your environment clutter-free and relatively organized can help minimize distractions and improve memory. For example, make a habit of always returning keys and handbags to a designated place. This makes it simple to find them next time.

organs in your body, the brain has a vast network of blood vessels that feed it the oxygen and nutrients necessary to operate successfully. As such, the brain also relies heavily on the heart's capacity to pump out the optimal amount of blood it needs.

Over time, the brain's vascular system begins to resemble that of the rest of the aging body — arteries in the brain become more narrow and less elastic, some become clogged with fatty deposits (a condition known as atherosclerosis), and the growth of new capillaries (offshoots from the main arteries) slows down.

Putting correspondence in order can help you stay on top of the endless stream of mail and paper that enters the home. It can also prevent unpaid bills and missed appointments. One method is to create different folders or places for: information that requires a response or action, such as bills or invitations; information that you'll need to consult occasionally, such as bank statements or insurance policies; and information to read at your leisure, such as magazines and catalogs.

FOCUS YOUR ATTENTION Attention is an important part of memory processing. It takes concentration to input information into your brain so that it can be stored and retrieved properly. Slow down and focus on the task at hand. Use your senses — sight, hearing, taste, touch and smell — to tune in to the present. Minimize distractions in order to provide your undivided attention to a person or project.

USE MEMORY TRICKS Memory tricks are creative techniques that prompt you to manipulate new information in a way that helps you recall it later. For example, repeating information out loud or associating mental images with names or facts can help you remember. Breaking up information into chunks is useful, too. Instead of remembering a grocery list of seven random items, think of the list as four vegetables and three fruits.

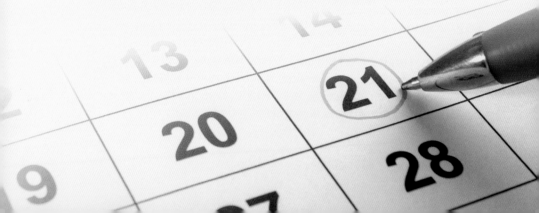

At the same time, the heart may not pump with its previous efficiency. As a result, the brain may receive a substandard amount of blood and the blood that does arrive may not flow through the brain as well as it once did.

This wear and tear on the brain's vascular system can result in microscopic injuries, inflammation and oxidative stress. In addition, the presence of other conditions such as high blood pressure, atherosclerosis or diabetes can further aggravate these effects on the brain's vascular system.

It's possible that a faulty, aging vascular system may create a brain environment that makes it easier for the destruction of nerve cells and communication pathways to occur. Various studies have linked cardiovascular risk factors in midlife — such as high blood pressure, high cholesterol and obesity — to later cognitive impairment and dementia.

Alzheimer's disease, the most common form of dementia, and cerebrovascular disease — such as stroke or mini-strokes, which themselves can cause brain injury and dementia (vascular cognitive impairment) — also frequently occur together. In fact, it's often difficult to separate one from the other.

The good news is that keeping your heart and blood vessels healthy will help keep your brain supplied with the right amount of blood it needs. It will also help keep blood flowing freely through your brain. Chapter 14 outlines specific strategies and practical suggestions to increase your heart health.

KEEP MOVING Physical activity can have brain benefits independent of the benefits it confers on your heart. Physical activity seems to help the brain not only by keeping your blood flowing but also by directly supporting the health of brain cells.

Animal and human studies indicate that aerobic exercise increases the release of a substance called brain-derived neurotrophic factor (BDNF). BDNF promotes neuron survival and growth, enhances the formation of connections between neurons, supports new blood vessel formation, and encourages generation of new neurons in the hippocampus, the key memory center of the brain.

Clinical studies also suggest that exercise appears to inhibit some Alzheimer's-like changes in the brain. Several studies in mice and in humans show an association between long-term exercise and lower levels of amyloid plaques in the brain. Amyloid plaques are abnormal structures that are a characteristic feature of Alzheimer's disease.

Evidence suggests that, in the short term, aerobic exercise improves various measures in cognitive testing, including memory, attention, processing speed, and judgment and decision-making. Exercise may also enhance the connectivity and activation of neurons.

In the long term, regular physical activity can reduce your risk of dementia. An analysis of multiple studies found that adults who routinely engaged in physical activities, sports or regular exercise during midlife had a significantly lower risk of dementia years later. Likewise, the risk of mild cognitive impairment, often considered a precursor to Alzheimer's disease, was reduced in women who reported exercising earlier in life. One study connected a program of regular walking with increased volume in the hippocampus, thus potentially countering age-related loss of brain volume and associated memory impairment.

Cross-train your brain

Just as you might exercise your body to gain physical strength, you can also exercise your brain to increase intellectual capacity. Early research suggests that brain training programs may improve your memory, mental processing speed and ability to perform everyday activities.

There's a wide range of available online brain training programs, computer software programs and smartphone apps with scientific merits at varying price points. These programs run you through various exercises, often on a timer, that gradually ramp up the level of difficulty so that your brain is continually stretched and challenged.

Of course, you can achieve much the same effect on your own by doing increasingly harder number games or more-complex crafts, for example. The key is to practice, practice, practice. Challenge yourself and target a range of skills — do jigsaw puzzles to sharpen spatial relationship skills and play speed card games with the neighbor's kid to increase mental processing speed, for example.

Most studies have focused on aerobic exercise — the kind that increases your heart rate and your need for oxygen — but it's possible that strength training and resistance exercise may help as well.

If your shoulders sag at the mention of aerobic exercise, keep in mind that this doesn't have to mean hours at the gym, necessarily, although that certainly won't hurt. The simplest aerobic exercise may be putting on your sneakers and walking, which can be done practically anytime, anywhere. But doing yardwork, dancing, cleaning (dancing while cleaning!), playing tennis or racquetball, or hiking — these all count too if you do them in a sustained manner. For brain benefits, aim for 30 minutes a day, most days of the week.

More research is needed to know to what degree adding physical activity improves memory or slows the progression of cognitive decline. Nonetheless, evidence so far strongly suggests that regular exercise is important to stay mentally fit.

BUILD UP YOUR RESERVE In addition to protecting your heart and staying physically fit, there's another factor that may play an important role in preserving your brain health. It involves the concept of cognitive reserve — essentially your brain's ability to adapt to age- or disease-related changes by drawing on existing neuronal networks or generating new neuronal connections where old ones may fail.

Your cognitive reserve relates to brain networks set up by factors such as brain size and neuron count, natural intelligence, life experience, education, and occupation. The greater your reserve, the more leeway your brain has when asked to perform certain tasks — something that becomes more important as time goes by.

The idea that you can increase your cognitive reserve is a hot topic in research these days. It implies the possibility of preventing or compensating for cognitive decline by strengthening nerve networks and even building new ones through intellectual and social stimulation.

Most studies show a positive link between having an active social and intellectual life throughout the adult years, and a decreased risk of cognitive impairment in later years.

A recent study by Mayo Clinic researchers offers a good example. The investigators found that ordinary yet intellectually stimulating activities such as using a computer, playing games, reading books and engaging in crafts — including knitting, woodworking and other types of handiwork — were associated with a 30 to 50 percent decrease in the chances of developing mild cognitive impairment.

As with physical exercise, some activities seem to provide more of a cognitive workout than others. For example, the Mayo study found that reading newspapers had less effect than reading books. In addition, watching less TV was more favorable for cognitive health than watching more. Other studies have mentioned taking courses, learning new languages, traveling and going to the theater, to name just a few. The important part may be choosing those activities that absorb your mind, draw you in and engage your thought processes.

It also may be that engaging in intellectually and socially stimulating activities helps reduce stress. For example, playing a game with another person usually involves a deliberate effort to pay attention to what you're doing. People who are working on a craft often find themselves becoming completely immersed in what they're doing.

This is similar in some ways to meditative techniques that focus on becoming fully aware of the here and now. Such techniques tend to produce a relaxation response — sort of the opposite of the body's fight-or-flight response to stress. The relaxation response decreases your blood pressure, heart rate and breathing rate. It increases concentration, immersion in the moment, and feelings of contentment and well-being. It may also help buffer areas of the brain from stress-related changes, thus preserving neurons and their connections.

Finally, participating in enjoyable leisure activities, especially social ones, can help prevent depression and loneliness, both of which have been associated with poor cognitive health.

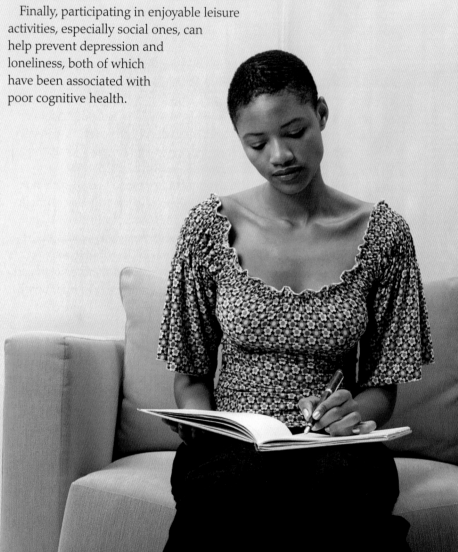

CHAPTER SIXTEEN

Taking care of your body

You know you've earned your stripes in the years leading up to menopause. But crow's-feet and a hairy upper lip — really? Chapter 3 outlined many of the common body changes that occur with menopause. Now it's time to look at what you can do to keep your body in its best operating shape throughout this next act of your life.

Earlier chapters have touched on important steps for overall health — namely the importance of a healthy diet, regular exercise and ample sleep. In this chapter, you'll learn about specific tips to care for the areas commonly affected by menopause, from your hair to your joints. With some maintenance efforts, some common menopausal changes may be preventable. And those that do occur can be minimized and managed. With some care, you might even find yourself healthier than ever in the years after menopause.

Care for changing hair

Your hair may have been your crowning glory in your teens and 20s. But these days, it's looking a little worse for wear. Or perhaps the problem is hair that's cropping up in the most unexpected — and annoying — of places.

Can anything be done? Absolutely.

AVOIDING DAMAGE Hair damage occurs when the protective fat (lipid) layer that makes hair shiny and pliable is destroyed. This gives hair a dried out, dull and frizzy appearance, and also makes hair more brittle and prone to breakage. To keep hair healthy, avoid damage caused by:

Chemical products Frequent coloring, relaxing or perms can damage your hair. A natural color and style involving minimal chemicals is optimal. Short of that, try to space colorings as far apart as possible. Avoid care involving coloring and a perm or relaxer at the same sitting.

Heat Too much heat can damage hair. Letting hair air-dry or going with your natural level of curliness is best. Short of that, use a hair dryer or curling iron on a low setting. With hair straighteners, place a moist cloth over the hot plates of the device so that they don't directly touch the hair.

Rough handling Straight, wavy or loosely curly hair breaks more easily when wet. Be gentle when towel-drying. Let hair become mostly dry before gently combing it with a wide-toothed comb. For those of African descent with tightly curled hair, combing hair while damp is preferred. Only comb as little as needed to style your hair.

Tight hairstyles Avoid prolonged wearing of hairstyles such as pony-tails, cornrows or braids.

Improper shampooing Massage shampoo into your scalp with your fingertips and rinse it away. After shampooing, use a conditioner on your hair if your hair tends to be dry or tangle easily.

THINNING HAIR SOLUTIONS If your hair seems to be pulling a disappearing act, you can thank the change in hormones. Still, there are options to explore:

Treat your hair gently Follow the steps above to prevent damage.

Eat a nutritionally balanced diet Poor nutrition can increase your risk of hair loss. Be sure you're getting a good mix of fruits, vegetables and sources of protein.

See your health care provider While the onset of menopause is often a common culprit for hair loss, it's not always the cause. Be sure to

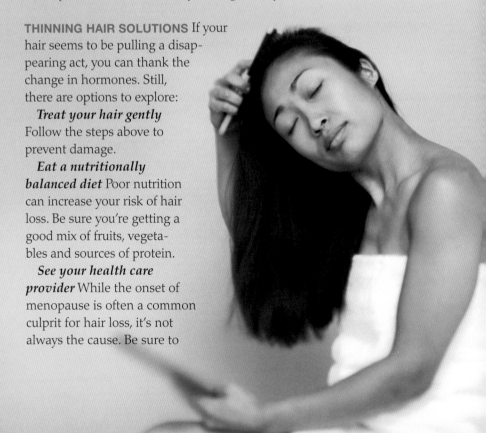

rule out any underlying health conditions or other causes before you explore treatments.

Consider minoxidil (Rogaine) Minoxidil is an over-the-counter liquid or foam that you rub into your scalp twice a day to grow hair and to prevent further hair loss. The effect peaks at 16 weeks, and you need to keep applying the medication to retain benefits. Possible side effects include scalp irritation, unwanted hair growth on the adjacent skin of the face and hands, and rapid heart rate (tachycardia).

Medications for unwanted hair

Medications usually take several months before you see a significant difference in hair growth. Medications may include:

▶ **Oral contraceptives.** Birth control pills or other hormonal contraceptives, which contain estrogen and a progestin, treat hair growth by decreasing androgens in a few different ways. Possible side effects include dizziness, nausea, headache and stomach upset.

▶ **Anti-androgens.** These types of drugs block sex hormones from attaching to their receptors in your body. The most commonly used anti-androgen for hair growth is spironolactone (Aldactone).

▶ **Topical cream.** Eflornithine (Vaniqa) is a prescription cream specifically for excessive facial hair in women. It's applied directly to the affected area of your face and helps slow new hair growth, but doesn't get rid of existing hair.

DEALING WITH UNWANTED HAIR Self-care measures to combat rogue body hair include:

Bleaching Instead of removing the hair, you may want to opt for using bleach to make it less visible. Bleach may cause skin irritation for some women, so be sure to test on a small area first.

Plucking The trusty tweezers. While plucking is a good method to remove a few stray hairs, it's not very practical for removing large areas of hair.

Shaving Shaving is quick and inexpensive, but it needs to be repeated regularly since it removes the hair only down to the surface of your skin.

Depilatory products These products are generally available as gels, lotions and creams that you spread on your skin. Chemical depilatories work by breaking down the protein structure of the hair shaft. It's a good idea to test a small patch of the product before applying on a larger area.

Wax Waxing involves applying warm wax on your skin where the unwanted hair grows. Once the wax hardens, it's pulled back from your skin against the direction of hair growth, removing hair. Waxing removes hair from a large area quickly, but it may sting temporarily and sometimes causes skin irritation and redness.

Laser hair removal During this procedure, a laser beam passes through the skin to an individual hair follicle. The intense heat of the laser damages the follicle, which inhibits future hair growth. However, it doesn't guarantee permanent hair removal. It typically takes multiple treatments, and periodic maintenance treatments might be needed as well. Laser hair removal is most effective for people who have light skin and dark hair.

Electrolysis This treatment involves inserting a tiny needle into each hair follicle. The needle emits a pulse of electric current to damage and eventually destroy the follicle. Electrolysis is an effective hair removal procedure, but it can be painful. A numbing cream spread on your skin before treatment may reduce this discomfort.

The eyes have it

The eyes are said to be the window to the soul. Keep those windows functioning their best with a little self-care.

HELP FOR DRY EYES As mentioned in Chapter 3, dry eyes are an especially common problem around the time of menopause — they're estimated to affect almost 3.25 million women age 50 and older. But it's not an issue you just have to grin and bear.

If you experience dry eyes, pay attention to the situations that are most likely to cause your symptoms. Then find ways to avoid those situations in order to prevent your dry-eye symptoms. For instance:

Avoid air blowing in your eyes Don't direct hair dryers, car heaters, air conditioners or fans toward your eyes.

Add moisture to the air A humidifier can add moisture to dry indoor air.

Consider wearing wraparound sunglasses or other protective eyewear Safety shields can be added to the tops and sides of eyeglasses to block wind and dry air. Ask about shields where you buy your eyeglasses.

Take eye breaks during long tasks If you're reading or doing another task that requires visual concentration, take periodic eye breaks. Close your eyes for a few minutes. Or blink repeatedly for a few seconds to help spread your tears evenly over your eyes.

Be aware of your environment The air at high altitudes, in desert areas and in airplanes can be extremely dry. When spending time in such an environment, it may be helpful to frequently close your eyes for a few minutes at a time to minimize evaporation of your tears.

Position your computer screen below eye level If your computer screen is above eye level, you'll open your eyes wider to view the screen. Position your computer screen below eye level so that you won't open your eyes as wide. This may help slow the evaporation of your tears between eye blinks.

Stop smoking and avoid smoke If you smoke, ask your health care provider for help devising a quit-smoking strategy that's most likely to work for you. Smoke can worsen dry-eye symptoms.

Choosing a dry-eye product

Consider these factors when selecting a nonprescription product for dry eyes:

▶ **Preservative versus nonpreservative drops.** Preservatives are added to some eyedrops to prolong shelf life. You can use eyedrops with preservatives up to four times a day. But using the preservative drops more often can cause eye irritation. Nonpreservative eyedrops come in packages that contain multiple single-use vials. After you use a vial, you throw it away. If you rely on eyedrops more than four times a day, nonpreservative drops may be safer.

▶ **Drops vs. ointments.** Lubricating eye ointments coat your eyes, providing long-lasting relief from dry eyes. But these products are thicker than eyedrops and can cloud your vision. Eyedrops can be used at any time and won't interfere with your vision.

▶ **Drops that reduce redness.** It's best to avoid these as your solution for dry eyes, as prolonged use can cause irritation.

If you've tried more than one product and are still not finding any relief, ask your health care provider about prescription medications and procedures that may be effective in your case.

Use artificial tears regularly If you have chronic dry eyes, use eyedrops to keep them well-lubricated even when your eyes feel fine. In addition to drops, there are gels, gel inserts and ointments available over-the-counter. See the sidebar, left, for tips on choosing the right product for you.

EVERYDAY EYE CARE Your overall eye health is important at any age. As you enter into an age where eye concerns become more common, here are tips for maintaining optimal vision:

Have regular eye examinations Eye exams can help detect eye problems at their earliest stages. As a general rule, have a comprehensive eye exam every four years beginning at age 40 and every two years from age 65. You may need more frequent screening if you're at high risk of eye disease or if you have corrected vision.

Know your family's eye health history Some eye diseases, such as glaucoma, tend to run in families.

Quit smoking Smoking puts you at risk of common eye conditions such as macular degeneration and cataracts. Ask your health care provider for suggestions about how to stop smoking. Medications, counseling and other strategies are available to help you.

Reduce alcohol use Excessive alcohol use can increase the risk of some eye problems.

Wear sunglasses Ultraviolet light from the sun may contribute to the development of cataracts. Wear sunglasses that block ultraviolet B (UVB) rays when you're outdoors.

Manage other health problems Follow your treatment plan if you have diabetes or other conditions that can increase your risk of eye disease.

Maintain a healthy weight Being overweight increases your risk of developing diabetes, high blood pressure and cardiovascular diseases. Each of these conditions can damage the small delicate vessels found in the eye and potentially lead to vision loss.

Choose a healthy diet that includes plenty of fruits and vegetables Adding a variety of colorful fruits and vegetables to your diet ensures that you're getting ample vitamins and nutrients. Fruits and vegetables have many antioxidants, which help maintain the health of your eyes.

Slowing hearing changes

Hearing loss that occurs gradually as you age is common. In fact, it's estimated that about 25 percent of people in the U.S. between the ages of

Eating for eye health

Did your mother ever tell you to finish your carrots because they were good for your eyes? Well, she was right.

The National Eye Institute and other vision experts note that a healthy diet is an important factor in eye health. Researchers have found that certain nutrients with antioxidant properties are beneficial — including beta carotene, lutein, zeaxanthin, and vitamins C and E. Zinc and omega-3 fatty acids also are important.

Here's a list of foods to include in your diet to help keep your eyes healthy:

▶ **Vegetables.** Kale, collard greens, peppers, broccoli, sweet potato, spinach, peas, pumpkin, carrots and Swiss chard

▶ **Fruits.** Peaches, blueberries, oranges, tangerines, mango, tomato, apricot, papaya, cantaloupe, honeydew, avocado and grapefruit

▶ **Sources of zinc.** King crab, lamb, bulgur, lean beef, fortified breakfast cereals, beans, lean pork, dark poultry meat, whole-wheat or buckwheat flours, pumpkin seeds

▶ **Omega-3-rich foods.** Salmon, herring, tuna, mackerel, rainbow trout, sardines, flaxseed, English walnuts, canola oil, roasted soybeans

55 and 64 have some degree of hearing loss. After age 65, that number creeps closer to 50 percent.

You can't reverse most types of hearing loss. But try not to speed up the process by putting yourself at risk from chronic noise exposure.

PROTECT YOUR EARS Here are steps you can take to prevent noise-induced hearing loss and avoid worsening age-related hearing loss:

Wear earplugs or earmuffs If you have to shout to be heard by someone an arm's length away, you're being exposed to too much noise. In such situations, wear protective earplugs or specially designed earmuffs that meet federal safety standards. This guideline applies at work and at home.

Manage recreational risks Activities such as riding a motorcycle or snowmobile, attending a rock concert, or firing a gun can damage your hearing. Wear hearing protection to blunt the noise. With the growing popularity of portable music players, experts expect more people will have hearing loss and at younger ages. Turning down the volume and setting volume limits on your devices can help you avoid damage.

Hold down the noise at home It's easy to overlook the daily racket. To reduce noise, control the volume on the TV and stereo, don't run multiple appliances at the same time, and when possible, purchase quieter appliances.

Have your hearing tested If you work in a noisy environment, have regular hearing tests. Testing can provide early detection of hearing loss so that you can take steps to prevent further damage to your hearing.

Showcase your smile

One of the best weapons you can have in your menopause arsenal is your smile. Are you keeping it healthy?

BRUSHING 101 Keeping the area where your teeth meet your gums clean can prevent gum disease, while keeping your tooth surfaces clean can help you stave off cavities. Consider these brushing basics:

Brush your teeth at least twice a day When you brush, don't rush. Take enough time to do a thorough job.

Use the proper equipment Use a fluoride toothpaste and a soft-bristled toothbrush that fits your mouth comfortably. Consider using an electric or battery-operated toothbrush, which can reduce plaque and a mild form of gum disease (gingivitis) more effectively than can manual brushing.

Practice good technique Hold your toothbrush at a slight angle — aiming the bristles toward the area where your tooth meets your gum. Gently brush with short back-and-forth motions. Remember to brush the outside, inside and chewing surfaces of your teeth, as well as your tongue.

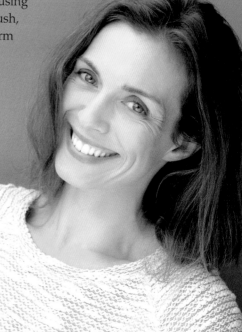

Keep your equipment clean Always rinse your toothbrush with water after brushing. Store your toothbrush in an upright position if possible and allow it to air-dry until using it again. Don't routinely cover toothbrushes or store them in closed containers, which can encourage the growth of bacteria.

Know when to replace your toothbrush Invest in a new toothbrush or a replacement head for your electric or battery-operated toothbrush every three to four months — or sooner if the bristles become frayed.

DON'T PASS ON THE FLOSS You can't reach the tight spaces between your teeth and under the gumline with a toothbrush. That's why daily flossing is important. When you floss:

Don't skimp Break off about 18 inches of floss. Wind most of it around the middle finger on one hand, and the rest around the middle finger on the other hand. Grip the floss tightly between your thumbs and forefingers.

Be gentle Guide the floss between your teeth using a rubbing motion. Don't snap the floss into your gums. When the floss reaches your gumline, curve it against one tooth.

Do one tooth at a time Slide the floss into the space between your gum and tooth. Use the floss to gently rub the side of the tooth in an up-and-down motion. Unwind fresh floss as you progress to the rest of your teeth.

Keep it up If you find it hard to handle floss, use an interdental cleaner — such as a special wooden or plastic pick, stick or brush designed to clean between the teeth.

SEE YOUR DENTIST To prevent gum disease and other oral health problems, schedule dental cleanings and exams at least once or twice a year.

Savor your skin

However young you may feel in spirit, your skin may be starting to tell a different story. As you age, your skin becomes drier and more lax and wrinkled — you'll likely lose about 30 percent of the collagen in your skin in the first five years after menopause. And you may start to notice more spots and growths, too.

You may not be able to change all your spots — or wrinkles. But proactive skin care can help keep your skin youthful and healthy.

PRACTICE SUN PROTECTION Start with skin care rule No. 1 — protect yourself from the sun.

Avoid the sun during peak hours Generally this is between 10 a.m. and 2 p.m., regardless of season. These are prime hours for exposure to skin-damaging ultraviolet (UV) radiation from the sun, even on overcast days.

Wear protective clothing This includes pants, shirts with long sleeves, wide-brimmed hats and sunglasses. Consider investing in sun-protective clothing or using an umbrella for shade. Laundry additives also are available, which give clothing an additional layer of ultraviolet protection.

Don't neglect sunscreen Apply generously and reapply regularly — generally every two hours, or even more often if you're swimming or perspiring. Use enough sunscreen to fully cover all bare skin, including your neck, face, ears, tops of your feet, back and legs.

Skip the tanning beds UV radiation damages your skin, whether the exposure comes from tanning beds or natural sunlight. In fact, tanning beds emit UVA rays — which might increase the risk of melanoma, the deadliest form of skin cancer.

Choosing a good sunscreen

No matter what stage of life you're in, using sunscreen can help prevent age-related skin changes and skin cancer. Choose a broad-spectrum sunscreen with a sun protection factor (SPF) of at least 15.

▶ A broad-spectrum, or full-spectrum, sunscreen is designed to protect you from two types of ultraviolet light that can harm your skin — UVA and UVB. SPF is a measure of how well a sunscreen deflects UVB rays.

▶ Remember to select a sunscreen that also protects against UVA. UVA rays may increase the risk of melanoma, the deadliest form of skin cancer.

DON'T SMOKE Smoking makes your skin look older and contributes to wrinkles. Smoking narrows the tiny blood vessels in the outermost layers of your skin, which decreases blood flow. This depletes the skin of oxygen and nutrients that are important to skin health. Smoking also damages collagen and elastin — the fibers that give your skin strength and elasticity.

If you smoke, the best way to protect your skin is to quit. Ask your health care provider for tips or treatments that can help.

A guide to anti-wrinkle products

Many wrinkle creams and lotions promise to reduce wrinkles and prevent or reverse damage caused by the sun. Do they work? That often depends on the specific ingredients and how long you use them.

If you're looking for a face-lift in a bottle, you probably won't find it in over-the-counter creams. But you may still experience modest benefits.

Common ingredients

The effectiveness of anti-wrinkle creams depends in part on the active ingredient or ingredients. Here are some common ingredients that may result in slight to modest improvement in the appearance of wrinkles.

▶ **Retinol.** Retinol is a vitamin A compound and an antioxidant. Antioxidants are substances that neutralize free radicals — unstable oxygen molecules that break down skin cells and cause wrinkles.

▶ **Vitamin C.** Another potent antioxidant, vitamin C may help protect skin from sun damage. Before and between uses, wrinkle creams containing vitamin C must be stored in a way that protects them from air and sunlight.

▶ **Hydroxy acids.** Alpha hydroxy acids, beta hydroxy acids and poly hydroxy acids are exfoliants — substances that remove the upper layer of old, dead skin and stimulate the growth of smooth, evenly pigmented new skin.

▶ **Coenzyme Q10.** This ingredient may help reduce fine wrinkles around the eyes and protect the skin from sun damage.

▶ **Tea extracts.** Green, black and oolong teas contain compounds with antioxidant and anti-inflammatory properties. Green tea extracts are the ones most commonly found in wrinkle creams.

▶ **Grape seed extract.** In addition to its antioxidant and anti-inflammatory properties, grape seed extract also promotes wound healing.

▶ **Niacinamide.** A potent antioxidant, this substance is related to vitamin B-3 (niacin). It helps reduce water loss in the skin and may improve skin elasticity.

No guarantees

The Food and Drug Administration (FDA) classifies creams and lotions as cosmetics, which are defined as having no medical value. So the FDA regulates them less strictly than it does drugs. This means that products don't undergo the same rigorous testing for safety and effectiveness that topically applied medications undergo before approval to go on the market.

Because the FDA doesn't evaluate cosmetic products for effectiveness, there's no guarantee that any over-the-counter product will reduce wrinkles. Consider these points when judging the merits of using a wrinkle cream:

▶ **Cost.** Cost has no relationship to effectiveness. A wrinkle cream that's more costly may not be more effective than a less costly product.

▶ **Lower doses.** Nonprescription wrinkle creams contain lower concentrations of active ingredients than do prescription creams. So results, if any, are limited and usually short-lived.

▶ **Multiplicity of ingredients.** There's no data to suggest that adding two or three of the earlier ingredients together will be more effective than just one of them.

▶ **Daily use.** You'll likely need to use the product once or twice a day for many weeks before noticing any improvements. And once you discontinue using the product, your skin is likely to return to its original appearance.

▶ **Side effects.** Some products may cause skin irritation, rashes, burning or redness. Be sure to read and follow the product instructions to limit possible side effects.

▶ **Individual differences.** Just because your friend swears by a product doesn't mean it will work for you. People have different skin types.

Your anti-wrinkle regimen

An anti-wrinkle cream may lessen the appearance of your wrinkles, depending on how often you use it, the type and amount of active ingredient, and the extent of the wrinkles you want to treat.

A dermatologist can help you create a personalized skin care plan by assessing your skin type, evaluating your skin's condition and recommending products likely to be effective. If you're looking for more dramatic results, a dermatologist can recommend medical treatments for wrinkles, including prescription creams, botulinum toxin (Botox) injections or skin-resurfacing techniques.

EAT A HEALTHY DIET A healthy diet can help you look and feel your best. Eat plenty of fruits, vegetables, whole grains and lean proteins. Some research suggests that a diet rich in vitamin C and low in unhealthy fats and processed or refined carbohydrates might promote younger looking skin.

MANAGE STRESS Uncontrolled stress can make your skin more sensitive and trigger acne breakouts and other skin problems. To encourage healthy skin, take steps to manage your stress. Set reasonable limits, scale back your to-do list and make time to do things you enjoy.

TREAT YOUR SKIN WELL Daily cleansing and shaving can take a toll on your skin. To keep it gentle:

Limit bath time Hot water and long showers or baths remove precious oils from your skin. Limit your time and use warm — not hot — water.

Avoid strong soaps They strip oil from your skin. Choose a mild cleanser.

Shave carefully To protect and lubricate your skin, apply shaving cream, lotion or gel before shaving. For the closest shave, use a clean, sharp razor. Shave in the direction the hair grows, not against it.

Pat dry After washing or bathing, gently pat or blot your skin dry with a towel so that some moisture remains on your skin.

Moisturize dry skin A good moisturizer includes a combination of ingredients that both hydrate the skin and hold water in the skin. Use a moisturizer that fits your skin type.

CONQUER ADULT ACNE It's not always a teenage problem, especially for women. Here's how to fight back:

Wash acne-prone areas only twice a day Washing removes excess oil and dead skin cells. But too much washing can irritate the skin. Wash affected areas with a gentle cleanser and use oil-free, water-based products.

Use an acne cream or gel to help dry excess oil Look for products containing benzoyl peroxide or salicylic acid as the active ingredient.

Use nonoily makeup Choose oil-free cosmetics, sunscreens and moisturizers that won't clog pores (noncomedogenic).

Remove makeup before going to bed Going to sleep with cosmetics on your skin can clog your pores. Also, it's a good idea to throw out old makeup and regularly clean your cosmetic brushes and applicators with soapy water.

Watch what touches your skin Keep your hair clean and off your face. Avoid resting your hands or objects on your face.

Shower after strenuous activities Oil and sweat left on your skin can lead to breakouts.

Don't neglect your joints

Your joints undergo a certain amount of wear and tear as you age. Protecting your joints is one of the most effective ways to avoid or relieve pain and prevent further joint damage. Follow the principles below to protect your joints from unnecessary strain.

RECOGNIZE AND ACKNOWLEDGE YOUR PAIN Learn to recognize the difference between general discomfort from a joint condition such as arthritis and pain from overuse of a joint. Then change your activity level or how you do a task to avoid excessive pain.

Pain that lasts more than an hour after an activity or exercise indicates the activity was too stressful. If you experience pain after an activity, consider the following factors, which may have contributed to the pain:

▶ What were you doing that involved the use of the painful joints?

▶ What position were you in?

▶ How long were you involved in the activity?

▶ Was the task too heavy or forceful?

The next time you're involved in the same activity, try changing one of these variables, and keep changing them (one at a time) until you learn what and how much your joint can do without causing pain.

PRACTICE CORRECT BODY MECHANICS Consider these ergonomic tips to protect your joints:

▶ When sitting, the proper height for a work surface is 2 inches below your bent elbow. Make sure you have good back and foot support when you sit. Your forearms and upper legs should be parallel with the floor.

▶ If you type at a computer or other keyboard for long periods and your chair doesn't have arms, consider using wrist or forearm supports. An angled work surface for reading and writing is easier on your neck.

▶ Increase the height of your chair seat to decrease the stress on your hips and knees as you get up and down.

Handling headaches

During perimenopause, when estrogen levels are swinging wildly as menstrual cycles become more erratic, migraines often get worse. Other menopausal symptoms — such as disrupted sleep, mood swings and hot flashes — may contribute to headaches, not just of migraine but tension-type and chronic daily headaches, as well.

For women with migraine, the good news is that once your final period occurs and estrogen levels smooth out, migraines often improve. The exception is for women who have migraine with aura, who may not experience the same type of relief with menopause. The arrival of menopause also doesn't seem to "cure" tension-type and chronic daily headaches.

If you experience a new headache — of any kind — during perimenopause or any other time, tell your health care provider. Together you can exclude other causes for headache as well as find the right type of relief.

Does hormone therapy help or hinder?

In some women, hormone therapy can worsen migraines, while in others it may ease them. It's important to talk to your health care provider about your individual circumstances and any kind of headache you have. Easing other symptoms of menopause may help with headache.

In general, experts recommend avoiding hormonal fluctuations if possible. In the time leading up to menopause, this might mean taking a hormonal contraceptive in a continuous rather than a cyclical regimen, or including a shortened hormone-free period.

Finding relief

Treatment for headaches during menopause is really no different from other times. If you have migraine, you'll want to avoid migraine triggers and take quick-relief medications — such as ibuprofen, acetaminophen-caffeine combinations or a prescription medication such as a triptan — as soon as you feel one coming on. In addition, your health care provider may have you on preventive medications — such as a beta blocker or calcium channel blocker — to decrease recurrences. Work with your health care provider to find the one that works best for you.

For tension-type headaches, nonprescription pain relievers such as nonsteroidal anti-inflammatory drugs are often effective. Keep in mind that overuse of pain relievers — more than twice a week, for example — can result in the development of chronic daily headaches. You might also consider nondrug therapies, which can be helpful. These might include stress management, relaxation therapy, acupuncture or biofeedback.

- When standing, the height of your work surface should enable you to work comfortably without stooping or reaching.

- To pick up items from the floor, stoop by bending your knees and hips. Or sit in a chair and then bend over.

- Carry heavy objects close to your chest, supported by your forearms.

- Maintain good posture. Poor posture causes uneven weight distribution and may strain your ligaments and muscles.

GIVE IT A REST Your joints need breaks just like the rest of you. Alternate light and moderate activities throughout the day. Work at a steady and deliberate pace — don't rush! Try to rest before you become fatigued or sore.

REDUCE EXCESS BODY WEIGHT Carrying extra body weight contributes to joint problems in several ways. It puts added stress on weight-bearing joints, such as your hips and knees. In addition, fat tissue produces proteins that may cause harmful inflammation in and around your joints, which may lead to osteoarthritis.

REMAIN ACTIVE In addition to helping you feel good and control your weight, exercise can help strengthen muscles that support your joints, reduce joint pain and help you maintain your mobility — when it's done right.

The main precaution to take is to protect your joints from further damage. Listen to your body — don't force a motion if you feel pain, and cut back on the intensity if your muscles ache long after the activity is over.

Low-impact activities such as cycling, swimming and moderate strength training place less stress on your joints. Follow these tips:

- Start easy and increase intensity gradually.

- Warm any bothersome joints with a heat source before exercise and apply ice to them after.

- Cross-train by alternating between a variety of flexibility, strengthening and aerobic exercises throughout the week.

- Use appropriate equipment, such as proper footwear or a well-adjusted bicycle.

CHAPTER SEVENTEEN

An ounce of prevention

....

You may be dreading that first colonoscopy that was put on your schedule for next month — they're going to do what, exactly? While the procedure itself may be less than appealing, it might help to look at this important screening exam as an opportunity to invest in your health.

As you approach menopause and move into a new stage in life, make prevention a priority. Rather than focusing only on treating illnesses as they pop up, prevention means taking steps in your daily life and with your routine health care to prevent these concerns in the first place, as well as to catch and treat important diseases and conditions at an early, more manageable stage.

Two important pillars to prevention are to eat a healthy diet and exercise regularly, as you learned about in Chapter 10. Additionally, prevention involves staying on top of routine screening tests and recommended vaccinations, which are the focus of this chapter.

Recommended screenings

Here's a look at routine screening tests that are recommended for women as they enter into midlife and beyond. Keep in mind that the recommended screening schedules are for women at average risk — if you're at increased risk of a particular condition, your health care provider will work with you to come up with a screening schedule that's appropriate for you.

BLOOD PRESSURE MEASUREMENT This test — using an inflatable cuff around your arm — measures the peak pressure your heart generates when pumping blood through your arteries (systolic pressure) and the amount of pressure in your arteries when your heart is at rest between beats (diastolic pressure).

What's the test for? This test is used to detect high blood pressure. If you have high blood pressure, the longer it goes undetected and untreated, the higher your risk of a number of diseases, including heart attack, stroke, heart failure, kidney damage and eye damage.

When and how often should you have it done? Have your blood pressure checked at least every two years. However, you'll likely have it checked every time you see a health care provider. If your blood pressure is elevated, your provider may recommend more-frequent testing. Testing is especially important if you are black, overweight or inactive or have a family history of the condition. These factors put you at increased risk of high blood pressure.

What do the numbers mean? An ideal or normal blood pressure for an adult of any age is 119 millimeters of mercury (mm Hg) over 79 mm Hg or lower. This is commonly written as 119/79 mm Hg.

Blood pressure numbers

Category	Top number (systolic)		Bottom number (diastolic)
Normal* blood pressure	Less than 120	*and*	Less than 80
Prehypertension	120 to 139	*or*	80 to 89
Stage 1 hypertension	140 to 159	*or*	90 to 99
Stage 2 hypertension	160 or higher	*or*	100 or higher

*Normal means the preferred range in terms of cardiovascular risk

†Numbers are expressed in millimeters of mercury (mm Hg)

Based on Chobanian AV, et al. Seventh report of the Joint National Committee on Prevention, Detection, Evaluation, and Treatment of High Blood Pressure. *Hypertension.* 2003;42:1206.

BREAST CANCER SCREENING Two tests — a clinical breast exam and mammogram — are typically done in conjunction with one another. A clinical breast exam (CBE) is a physical check of your breasts and underarms that's typically part of a routine physical. With a mammogram, images are taken of your breast tissue while your breasts are compressed between X-ray plates.

What's the test for? To detect cancer and precancerous changes in the breasts. With a CBE, your health care provider examines your breasts looking for lumps, color changes, skin irregularities and changes in your nipples. He or she then feels for enlarged lymph nodes under your arms. A mammogram can help point out small breast lumps and calcifications — often the first indication of early-stage breast cancer — which are too small to be detected on a physical exam.

When and how often should you have it? Before age 40, women should have a CBE at least every three years. For women age 40 and older, the exam is best done every year. Having regular breast exams is particularly important if you have a family history of breast cancer or other factors, including advancing age, which puts you at increased risk of breast cancer.

As outlined in Chapter 12, there's been disagreement in recent years over the best screening schedule for mammograms. At Mayo Clinic, the current practice is to recommend an annual screening mammogram beginning at age 40. Talk with your health care provider about a schedule that's right for you. Chapter 12 also outlines other breast imaging methods that may be used in addition to a mammogram.

CERVICAL CANCER SCREENING With a Pap test, your health care provider inserts a plastic or metal speculum into your vagina to view the cervix. Then, using a spatula and a soft brush, he or she gently obtains scrapings from the cervix, places the sample in a bottle, and sends it to a laboratory for analysis. This test may be accompanied by human papillomavirus (HPV) screening, which involves the same process and can be done at the same time as the Pap test.

What's the test for? The Pap test detects cancer and precancerous changes in the cervix. HPV screening is done to check for the presence of a high-risk strain of HPV. Almost all cervical cancers are linked to infection with a high-risk strain of this sexually transmitted virus.

When and how often should you have it? Women should start having Pap tests at age 21. For women ages 21 to 29, Pap tests are recommended every three years. Women over age 30 should have a Pap test every three years, or co-testing — HPV testing in addition to the Pap test — every five years. In some cases, the HPV test may be done on its own.

For women who've had a total hysterectomy — which includes removal of the cervix — for a noncancerous condition, routine Pap tests aren't necessary.

They're also not necessary if you're age 65 or older, you've had normal test results over the past 10 years (including the last three Pap tests or the last two co-tests), and you aren't at high risk of developing cervical cancer. When in doubt, ask your health care provider what's appropriate for you.

Regular Pap tests are especially important if you smoke or have had a sexually transmitted infection or multiple sex partners or if you have a history of cervical, vaginal or vulvar cancer. You're also at increased risk of cervical cancer and should be screened regularly if your immune system is suppressed or you were exposed to the synthetic hormone diethylstilbestrol (DES) in utero.

Although there's no known cure for HPV infection, the cervical changes that result from it can be treated. Fortunately, for most women, HPV infection clears on its own within one to two years.

CHOLESTEROL TEST A blood cholesterol test is actually made up of several blood tests. It measures total cholesterol in your blood, as well as levels of low-density lipoprotein (LDL), or "bad," cholesterol, high-density lipoprotein (HDL), or "good," cholesterol and other blood fats called triglycerides.

What's the test for? To measure the levels of cholesterol and triglycerides (lipids) in your blood. Undesirable lipid levels raise your risk of heart attack and stroke. Problems occur when your LDL cholesterol contributes to fatty deposits (plaques) developing on your artery walls or when your HDL cholesterol carries away too little LDL cholesterol from the arteries.

When and how often should you have it? Have a cholesterol evaluation at least every five years if the levels are within normal ranges. If the readings are abnormal, have your cholesterol checked more often. Cholesterol testing is especially important if you have a family history of high cholesterol or heart disease, are overweight, are physically inactive, or have diabetes. These factors put you at increased risk of developing high cholesterol and heart disease.

What do the numbers mean? The National Cholesterol Education Program has established guidelines to help determine which numbers are acceptable and which carry increased risk. However, desirable ranges vary, depending on your individual health conditions, habits and family history. Talk with your health care provider about what cholesterol levels are best for you and what you can do to achieve and maintain them.

COLORECTAL CANCER SCREENING For this screening exam, a variety of tests may be used. You may have just one or a combination.

Basic cholesterol guidelines

While individual cholesterol goals may vary, here's a breakdown of general cholesterol guidelines.

Total cholesterol

Below 200 milligrams per deciliter (mg/dL)	Desirable
200-239 mg/dL	Borderline high
240 mg/dL and above	High

LDL cholesterol

Below 100 mg/dL	Optimal
100-129 mg/dL	Near optimal
130-159 mg/dL	Borderline high
160-189 mg/dL	High
190 mg/dL and above	Very high

HDL cholesterol

Below 50 mg/dL (for women)	Poor
50-59 mg/dL	Better
60 mg/dL and above	Best

Triglycerides

Below 150 mg/dL	Desirable
150-199 mg/dL	Borderline high
200-499 mg/dL	High
500 mg/dL and above	Very high

Based on NCEP Expert Panel. Third report of the National Cholesterol Education Program (NCEP) Expert Panel on Detection, Evaluation, and Treatment of High Blood Cholesterol in Adults (Adult Treatment Panel III) final report. *Circulation.* 2002;106:3143.

- **Colonoscopy.** With this exam, a long, flexible tube (colonoscope) is inserted into the rectum, which allows the health care provider to examine the entire length of your colon. This is considered the gold standard for colon cancer screening.

- **Virtual colonoscopy.** For this exam, computerized tomography (CT) is used to produce cross-sectional images of your abdominal organs.

- **Flexible sigmoidoscopy.** Similar to a colonoscopy, a thin tube is inserted into your rectum. However, this test only evaluates the lower part of the colon (sigmoid colon).

- **Barium enema.** For this test, an X-ray is taken of your colon after you have an enema with a white, chalky substance that outlines the colon (barium X-ray).

- **Fecal occult blood test or fecal immunochemical test.** With these tests, a stool sample is tested in a lab for hidden (occult) blood.

- **Stool DNA test.** This test uses a stool sample to look for DNA changes in cells that might indicate the presence of colon cancer or precancerous conditions. It also looks for signs of blood in your stool.

What's the test for? To detect cancer and precancerous growths (polyps) on the inside of the wall of the colon that could become cancerous. Many people are afraid to have colorectal cancer screening because of fear of embarrassment or worry or discomfort. However, this screening could save your life by detecting precancerous polyps that can be removed, preventing this common cancer from occurring. Early detection of cancer also can be lifesaving.

When and how often should you have it? If you're at average risk of developing colorectal cancer, have a screening test every three to 10 years, beginning at age 50. The frequency of screening will depend on the type of test you have. If you have a personal or family history of colorectal cancer or polyps, you will require more-frequent screening.

Talk with your health care provider about which screening approach and frequency are best for you, given your particular health issues. If you're at increased risk of developing colorectal cancer, he or she may recommend beginning screenings at an earlier age and scheduling them more frequently.

DENTAL CHECKUP Your dentist examines your teeth and checks your tongue, lips, mouth and soft tissues.

What's the test for? A dental exam is done to detect tooth decay, problems such as tooth grinding and diseases such as gum (periodontal) disease. Your dentist also looks for lesions and other abnormalities in your mouth that could indicate cancer.

When and how often should you have it? Have a dental checkup every six months to one year, or as your dentist recommends. Regular dental checkups are especially important if your drinking water doesn't contain fluoride or if you use tobacco, regularly drink alcoholic or high-sugar beverages, or eat foods that are high in sugar.

DIABETES SCREENING Two blood tests are commonly used to screen for diabetes. A fasting blood sugar test measures the level of sugar (glucose) in your blood after an eight-hour fast. An A1C test measures your average glucose level over the last two or three months by measuring what percentage of your hemoglobin — a protein in red blood cells that carries oxygen — is coated with sugar.

What's the test for? Diabetes screening can detect high (elevated) glucose levels, which can cause damage to your heart and circulatory system.

When and how often should you have it? Have a baseline screening by age 45. If your results are normal, have your blood sugar rechecked every three years. If you have a family history of diabetes or other risk factors for the disease, such as obesity, your health care provider may recommend that you be tested at a younger age and more frequently. Screening is also recommended if you have signs and symptoms of diabetes, such as excessive thirst, frequent urination, unexplained weight loss, fatigue, or slow-healing cuts or bruises.

What do the numbers mean? A normal blood glucose level for an adult of any age is 70 to 99 milligrams per deciliter (mg/dL). If your blood sugar is between 100 and 125 mg/dL, you're considered to have prediabetes. Prediabetes is a medical condition that puts you at a higher risk of developing diabetes in the future. If your blood sugar is equal to or greater than 126 mg/dL on two separate tests, you'll be diagnosed with diabetes. For someone who doesn't have diabetes, a normal A1C level is below 5.7 percent, while an A1C between 5.7 and 6.4 percent indicates prediabetes. An A1C of 6.5 percent or higher on two separate tests indicates that you have diabetes.

EYE EXAM During an eye exam, you read eye charts and have your pupils dilated with eyedrops. Your health care provider also views the inside of your eye with an instrument called an ophthalmoscope and checks the pressure inside your eye with a painless procedure called tonometry.

What's the test for? An eye exam allows your ophthalmologist or optometrist to check your vision and determine whether you may be at risk of developing vision problems.

When and how often should you have it? If you wear glasses or contact lenses, have your eyes checked once a year. If you don't wear corrective lenses and have no risk factors for eye disease, have your eyes checked every two to four years until age 65. After age 65, it's best to have an exam every year or two.

Diabetes screening numbers

	Blood sugar level	AIC
Normal	70 to 99 milligrams per deciliter (mg/dL)	Below 5.7 percent
Prediabetes*	100 to 125 mg/dL	5.7 to 6.4 percent
Diabetes	126 mg/dL or higher on two separate tests	6.5 percent or higher on two separate tests

*Prediabetes means that your blood sugar level is higher than normal, but it's not yet high enough to be classified as type 2 diabetes. Still, without intervention, prediabetes is likely to become type 2 diabetes in 10 years or less.

HEARING TEST During a hearing test, a hearing specialist (audiologist) or other health care provider checks how well you recognize speech and sounds at various volumes and frequencies.

What's the test for? To check for hearing loss, which becomes more common with increased age.

When and how often should you have it? Have your hearing checked every 10 years until age 50. Starting at age 50, have it checked every three years. Hearing tests are especially important if you have been exposed to loud noises through your job or recreational activities, have had frequent ear infections, or are older than age 60. These factors increase your risk of hearing loss.

OSTEOPOROSIS SCREENING Bone density is measured by way of a specialized X-ray scan of a few bones — usually in the hip and spine.

What's the test for? To detect osteoporosis — a disease most common to women that involves gradual loss of bone mass, making your bones more fragile and likely to fracture. Osteoporosis most often increases the risk of fractures of the hip, spine and wrist. There are several different types of scans available. They include dual energy X-ray absorptiometry (DXA) and computerized tomography (CT). These tests are described in detail in Chapter 14.

Hepatitis C testing for baby boomers

The Centers for Disease Control and Prevention (CDC) recommends that women (and men) born between the years 1945 and 1965 get a one-time blood test for hepatitis C.

Hepatitis C is a liver disease resulting from infection with the hepatitis C virus. This disease can lead to serious health problems, including liver damage, cirrhosis of the liver and liver cancer.

For reasons still unknown, baby boomers are five times more likely than other adults to be infected with hepatitis C. However, there are treatments available if the disease is detected.

Women born after 1965 aren't included in this recommendation. However, if you have other risk factors for hepatitis C — such as receiving blood or an organ transplant before 1992 or having a history of high-risk sexual behavior — ask a health care professional about screening.

When and how often should you have it? Women should have a baseline exam at age 65. However, if you have a family history of osteoporosis or other risk factors, earlier testing is a good idea. Risk factors for osteoporosis include early menopause, frequent or extended use of steroid medications, smoking, excessive alcohol consumption, low body weight, rheumatoid arthritis, and a history of fractures.

What do the numbers mean? The T-score is a number that describes how much your bone density varies from what's considered "normal." Normal is based on the typical bone mass of women in their 30s — the period of life when bone mass is at its peak. Peak bone mass varies from one person to another and is influenced by many factors, including heredity, sex and race. Men tend to have higher bone mass than do women, and whites and Asians generally have lower bone density than do blacks and Hispanics.

- A T-score above -1.0 means that your bone density is considered normal. And you're at low risk of bone fractures.

- A T-score ranging from -1 to -2.5 indicates you have relatively low bone mass.

- A T-score of -2.5 and lower indicates you have osteoporosis and are at greater risk of bone fractures.

SEXUALLY TRANSMITTED INFECTION SCREENING Sexually transmitted infections (STIs), such as chlamydia and gonorrhea, are not just a problem for the college scene. And often, these infections don't show symptoms in the early stages.

What's the test for? To determine the presence of STIs, which are generally acquired by sexual contact. The organisms that cause these infections may pass from person to person in blood, semen, or vaginal and other body fluids. Apart from HPV screening — which is discussed with cervical cancer screening — STI screening is not routine for women in midlife. But if you're engaging in unprotected sex or you have multiple partners, screening is important.

When and how often should you have it? Before having intercourse with a new partner, be sure you've both been tested for STIs. It's recommended that you have at least one HIV screening during your lifetime, but more may be appropriate if you engage in behaviors that increase your risk, such as having unprotected sex and having sexual contact with multiple partners.

SKIN EXAMINATION In this exam, your health care provider examines your skin from head to toe, looking for moles and spots that are irregularly shaped, have varied colors, are asymmetrical, are greater than the size of a pencil eraser, bleed or have changed since the previous visit.

What's the test for? To check for signs of skin cancer, or other skin changes that may put you at increased risk of skin cancer.

When and how often should you have it? Consider having a full-body skin exam annually once you turn 50. Regular screening for skin cancer is especially important if you have many moles, fair skin, sun-damaged skin or a family history of skin cancer or if you've had two or more blistering sunburns in childhood or adolescence. These factors put you at increased risk of developing skin cancer. It's also important to check your own skin for changes, preferably once a month.

Preventive screening exams for women

These recommendations are based on average risk and normal results on prior testing.

Type of screening	Ages 50 to 59
Blood pressure	At least every 2 years
Breast cancer	Every 1-2 years
Cervical cancer	Every 3-5 years
Cholesterol	At least every 5 years
Colorectal cancer	Every 3-10 years (depends on test)
Diabetes	Every 3 years
Eye health	Every 2-4 years; annually if you wear glasses or contacts
Hearing	Every 3 years
Osteoporosis	Ask health care provider
Sexually transmitted infections	Every year if at increased risk; at least one lifetime HIV screening
Skin	Ask health care provider

Recommended vaccinations

One of the best ways to prevent many diseases is to make sure you've received all of the recommended vaccinations. Vaccines work by stimulating your body's natural defense mechanisms to resist infectious disease,

Ages 60 to 69	Ages 70 to 79	Ages 80 and older
At least every 2 years	At least every 2 years	At least every 2 years
Every 1-2 years	Every 1-2 years	Ask health care provider
Every 3-5 years; ask health care provider after age 65	Ask health care provider	Ask health care provider
At least every 5 years	At least every 5 years	At least every 5 years
Every 3-10 years (depends on test)	Every 3-10 years (depends on test). Ask health care provider after age 75	Ask health care provider
Every 3 years	Every 3 years	Every 3 years
Until age 65, every 2-4 years; beginning at age 65, every 1-2 years; annually if you wear glasses	Every 1-2 years; annually if you wear glasses or contacts	Every 1-2 years; annually if you wear glasses or contacts
Every 3 years	Every 3 years	Every 3 years
Baseline by age 65	Ask health care provider	Ask health care provider
Every year if at increased risk; at least one lifetime HIV screening	Every year if at increased risk; at least one lifetime HIV screening	Every year if at increased risk; at least one lifetime HIV screening
Ask health care provider	Ask health care provider	Ask health care provider

destroying the disease-causing microbes before you become sick. Most vaccinations are given in childhood. But there are some vaccines that are recommended specifically for adults or may be recommended regularly throughout life. Or it may be that you didn't receive a vaccination in childhood, which, if given now, still could be of benefit.

When in doubt, follow your health care provider's advice on which vaccinations to receive and when. He or she may recommend additional vaccinations depending on your occupation, hobbies or travel plans.

CHICKENPOX (VARICELLA) This viral disease spreads easily from person to person. Chickenpox is much more serious in adults than in children.

When you're at increased risk You're a health care worker without immunity or an adult who has never been exposed to the disease or never been vaccinated.

Doses for adults A two-dose series is given four to eight weeks apart. Avoid this if you have weakened immunity or lymph node or bone marrow cancer or if you've had a serious allergic reaction to gelatin or the antibiotic neomycin.

HEPATITIS A A viral infection of the liver transmitted primarily through contaminated food or water or close personal contact.

When you're at increased risk You are traveling to a country without clean water or proper sewage, you have chronic liver disease or a blood-clotting disorder, or you use illegal drugs

Doses for adults A two-dose series is given with at least six months between doses. Avoid this vaccination if you're hypersensitive to alum or 2-phenoxyethanol, a preservative.

HEPATITIS B A viral infection of the liver that's often transmitted through contaminated blood, sexual contact and prenatal exposure.

When you're at increased risk Your occupation puts you at risk of exposure to blood and body fluids, you have chronic liver disease, you are on dialysis or have received blood products, or you're sexually active with multiple partners.

Doses for adults A three-dose series is given during a six-month period to prevent the disease. Avoid this if you're allergic to baker's yeast.

INFLUENZA (FLU) A respiratory disease that spreads from person to person when you inhale infected droplets in the air.

When you're at increased risk You are age 50 or older, have a chronic disease or a weakened immune system, work in health care, or have close contact with people who are at high risk of the disease.

Doses for adults One dose every year is recommended for all adults. The vaccine is typically available as an injection or as a nasal spray. If you're age 65 or older, consider receiving the high-dose version of the vaccine. Talk to your health care provider if you're allergic to eggs or if you've had a previous reaction to a flu shot — some preparations may be available that are less likely to cause an allergic reaction.

MEASLES, MUMPS AND RUBELLA These are viral diseases that spread from person to person when infected droplets in the air are inhaled.

When you're at increased risk You were born after 1956 and don't have proof of previous vaccination or immunity.

Doses for adults One or two doses are given. Avoid this if you received blood products in the past 11 months, have weakened immunity or are allergic to the antibiotic neomycin.

MENINGOCOCCAL DISEASE A disease caused by bacteria that can cause meningitis, an inflammation of the membranes surrounding the brain and spinal cord.

When you're at increased risk You have a compromised immune system or you travel to certain foreign countries.

Doses for adults A single dose can prevent a bacterial form of the illness.

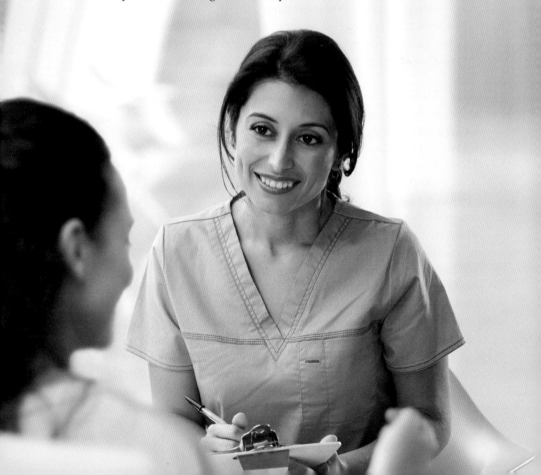

If you travel internationally

If you're planning to travel out of the country, make sure you're up to date on routine vaccinations, such as those for tetanus, diphtheria, pertussis, influenza, measles, mumps and rubella. Also, depending on your destination, length of stay and medical history, you may need additional vaccines.

The Centers for Disease Control and Prevention (CDC) recommends that international travelers consider the following additional vaccinations:

▶ **Japanese encephalitis.** This vaccination is recommended if you will be traveling to rural areas in the Far East, Southeast Asia or the Asian subcontinent for four weeks or more.

▶ **Polio.** A single dose of this vaccine is recommended if you didn't have a polio booster as an adult and are traveling to Africa, Southeast Asia, the South Pacific islands, the Middle East, the Asian subcontinent, Eastern Europe or one of the former republics of the Soviet Union.

▶ **Typhoid.** This vaccination is recommended if you're traveling outside of the U.S., except to Australia, New Zealand, Western Europe or Canada.

▶ **Yellow fever.** This vaccination is recommended if you're traveling to certain parts of Africa, the Caribbean, Central America or South America.

See your health care provider at least four to six weeks before your departure to schedule the vaccinations you need. Some vaccinations require several injections spaced days or weeks apart. For more information, visit the CDC's website at *www.cdc.gov/travel.*

PNEUMONIA An infection of the lungs, which can have various causes, such as bacteria or viruses.

When you're at increased risk You're age 65 or older, you have a medical condition that increases your risk, such as chronic lung, liver or kidney disease, or you don't have a spleen or it's damaged.

Doses for adults There are currently two types of pneumococcal vaccines, which are recommended for all adults age 65 or older, with at least one year between the two. They may also be recommended for adults under age 65 with certain risk factors

TETANUS AND DIPHTHERIA (MAY INCLUDE PERTUSSIS) Tetanus is a bacterial infection that develops in deep wounds. Diphtheria is a bacterial infection contracted when you inhale infected droplets. Whooping cough (pertussis) causes upper respiratory symptoms and a hacking cough.

When you're at increased risk You experienced a deep or dirty cut or wound. For pertussis, you're at risk if you haven't received a previous pertussis vaccination — especially if you have close contact with an infant, for whom pertussis is particularly risky.

Doses for adults An initial tetanus and diphtheria (Td) series is given with a booster every 10 years. If your most recent booster was more than five years ago, get a booster within 48 hours after a wound. Tetanus, diphtheria and pertussis (Tdap) also is given as an initial three-dose series if you didn't finish the Td series as a child. Otherwise, get one dose of Tdap when you're due for a Td booster, followed by a Td booster every 10 years.

HERPES ZOSTER (SHINGLES) A viral infection that causes a painful rash. It's caused by varicella-zoster — the same virus that causes chickenpox.

When you're at increased risk You're older than age 50 and you have had chickenpox.

Doses for adults A single dose is given, generally recommended at age 60 or older — although the vaccine is approved for adults age 50 or older. Avoid this if you have a weakened immune system or are allergic to gelatin or the antibiotic neomycin. Also avoid the vaccine if you're receiving treatment with steroids, radiation or chemotherapy.

Partner with your provider

Keep in mind that the screening and vaccination recommendations in this chapter are general guidelines. Work with your health care provider to develop a schedule that fits your individual risks and preferences. Developing a healthy partnership with your provider — one where you can candidly discuss your risks, concerns and symptoms — is a key step in maintaining good health.

CHAPTER EIGHTEEN

Embracing the image in the mirror

Menopause is a very good problem to have. Until about 1900, women didn't have a life expectancy past the natural age of menopause. There was no such thing as a senior discount or a silver fox and no debate about whether gray hair is the new black. There was no expectation of growing old gracefully or golfing through your golden years. There was little chance that you could see your grandbaby graduate from high school or pose for a family photograph with four generations.

Unfortunately, today's society has collectively, conveniently forgotten these facts. Instead, a fictitious standard of beauty has been adopted for women over age 50 — one that bears no resemblance to how women age naturally. Like many, you may have deluded yourself into wondering why you can't have hard-earned wisdom and rock-hard abs all at the same time.

If you're struggling to embrace your menopausal self in the mirror, it's really no wonder. Menopause is a time of unbelievable change, and it takes a while to get comfortable in your new (old) skin. Plus, there are very few true depictions of this stage of life in the media to help guide or reassure you. Most of the women featured in magazines or movies are much younger or hiding behind a pair of Spanx and a team of makeup and photo-editing artists.

It's perfectly normal to feel self-conscious or embarrassed about some of the changes that occur during menopause. It's not shallow or silly if you struggle to accept some of the things that are happening to your body. This chapter gives you some practical ideas for finding a realistic, positive perspective and being kind to yourself — at least most of the time.

Aging versus menopause

Aging and menopause go hand in hand. So it can be difficult to tease them apart and determine which physical and mental changes stem from the natural aging process and which are directly linked to a decline in estrogen.

For the most part, it doesn't really matter. But it can be helpful to understand what natural aging really looks like. Improvements in health care and changes in the environment have significantly slowed the aging process over time, but a 60-year-old woman still isn't going to look like a 20-year-old model. Even 49-year-old Cindy Crawford doesn't look like 20-year-old Cindy Crawford. The truth is that the natural aging process simply isn't all that glamorous, despite all of the airbrushed images of older women that you've seen over the years.

Aging differs. There's no single, chronological timetable that all women follow. Genetics, lifestyle and disease affect the rate at which you age.

However, there are some normal changes that occur with healthy aging — even in the absence of any serious condition or disease. It's normal to gain some weight with age, especially around the waist. It's normal to lose some hearing with age, even if you have no evidence of hearing disorders or noise-induced hearing loss. You may also notice that you have trouble falling asleep or staying asleep, learning new things, or remembering familiar words or names. The normal aging process also affects your eyes, your teeth and gums, and your skin.

The human mind has an innate instinct to focus on imperfection, so if one thing is not right it can pull your attention like a magnet. During the aging process, it's natural for women to find some physical imperfection to zero in on. It might be your less-than-perky breasts, your thick waist, your "turkey neck," your spotted hands, your thin lips or your wrinkled knees. This is common and normal, but it's certainly not productive.

Remind yourself that every age is a package deal — you get something and you lose something. You don't gain wisdom without a few wrinkles. You can't be discerning and perceptive without a few scars or spots. In the end, these trade-offs are worth it.

Aging with gratitude

Gratitude represents your thankfulness for every experience, because each step of life can help you grow — sometimes materially, but almost always emotionally and spiritually. According to research, a daily practice of gratitude can boost your energy, improve your mood, generate optimism, enhance your well-being and self-esteem, and much more. During menopause and beyond, gratitude can help you gracefully accept the things that you cannot change. And this is one of the keys to successful aging.

An occasional grateful thought is helpful. But your goal is to make it a habit. Here are some ideas for sprinkling gratitude throughout your day:

▶ **Start your day with gratitude.** Before you even get out of bed, let your first thought be one of gratitude. Start with a few deep breaths and then think about five people in your life you're grateful for. While breathing in slowly and deeply, choose one of these people and bring that person's face in front of your closed eyes. Try to "see" this person as clearly as you can. Then send him or her silent gratitude while breathing out, again slowly and deeply. Repeat this exercise with all five. This practice will help you focus on what's most important in your life and provide context to your day.

▶ **Start a gratitude journal.** As you close your day, write at least one thing you're thankful for — your morning yoga class, lunch with a girlfriend, your daughter's smile, the fact that your computer didn't crash during an important meeting. Gratitude can be used for your body image as well — if you think about it, there's much about your body to be grateful for. Be as specific as possible. On a rough day, refer back to this journal for some respite from negative feelings.

▶ **Collect gratitude sayings.** You'll find poignant quotes about gratitude in many novels, great speeches and spiritual texts. When you stumble across a saying that you like, write it down. You can place quotes in antique frames and display them at your house or office. Or you can simply jot quotes on Post-it notes and hang them on your refrigerator, corkboard or car visor. When you have a bad day, call on these grateful thoughts to redirect your mind.

▶ **Be grateful to those you help.** Say thanks to people who seek your help. At this stage in life, your wisdom and unconditional love are a gift to others. Be grateful that you can share these gifts with others.

▶ **Look for the positives in the negatives.** Focusing on the positive doesn't mean you overlook a problem. It means you take a compassionate stance. Take hot flashes, for example. They're no fun. But, without them, you wouldn't be enjoying so many delicious lemon ice pops. And you may not have discovered your favorite new air-conditioned bookstore. And your grandson wouldn't have made that hilarious comment about your red face. And you wouldn't have laughed so hard over hot-flash stories and wine with your best girlfriends. This is the silver lining.

Which gratitude ideas might work for you? Feel free to adapt these strategies to fit into your life and your routine. For instance, if you already start your day with an early-morning jog and a cup of coffee, try practicing gratitude in the shower. Let the hot water overhead be your cue to send gratitude to five people or five things. Experiment with all of these ideas until gratitude becomes second nature.

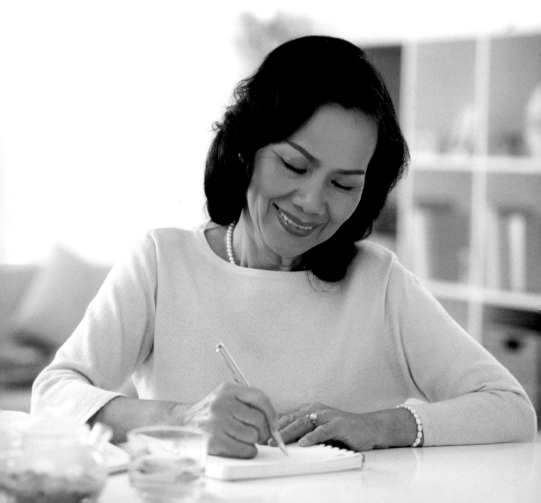

Your 40s, 50s and 60s are a very wise, productive time of life, when women typically feel very settled and confident at work and in their relationships. So you have a choice: You can be a harsh judge of the wrinkling woman in the mirror and make yourself miserable by squeezing your body into a pair of skinny jeans that's a size too small. Or you can focus on taking advantage of the opportunities and wisdom that you have earned.

Yes, some parts of the aging and menopause process are a drag. But it's important to see the blessings that come with growing older in addition to the blemishes. This act of acknowledging and appreciating your blessings is called gratitude (see pages 296-297).

Preventable versus inevitable changes

Let's just be clear: Your goal is to gracefully accept the changes that come with normal aging, not to accelerate your own decline by throwing in the towel.

Remember, normal aging and disease are distinct. Your body will naturally change with age. But adding candles to your birthday cake doesn't inevitably lead to disease. As you learned in earlier chapters, there are several keys to reducing your risk of the diseases and disabilities that can occur with age. Here's a recap:

MAINTAIN A HEALTHY WEIGHT As you know, many health problems are linked with being overweight or obese. This includes type 2 diabetes, high blood pressure, heart disease, stroke, some types of cancer, sleep apnea and osteoarthritis.

Since most people tend to gain some weight with age, it's important to keep an eye on your waistline and your body mass index (BMI). A couple of extra pounds may be OK. But a couple of extra pounds every year will be significant over the long haul. Focus on maintaining a healthy weight, not necessarily your premenopausal weight, and commit to making it happen. Being overweight is a serious health risk.

GET REGULAR PHYSICAL ACTIVITY Research suggests that people who exercise regularly actually live longer and live better. Staying active can also help you continue to do the things that you enjoy and stay independent as you age. Choose a well-rounded physical activity program that includes balance exercises, flexibility or stretching exercises, and strength training in addition to cardio time.

EAT A HEALTHY DIET What you eat can either support healthy aging or cause health problems. Of course, eating a healthy diet will help you maintain a healthy weight. But your food choices are important in other ways as you age, too. Eating unhealthy foods may increase your risk of some diseases. In contrast, eating well can help protect you from age-related problems caused by deficiencies of certain micronutrients and vitamins.

BE TOBACCO-FREE As you learned earlier in this book, it's never too late to enjoy the benefits of quitting smoking. There are clear benefits to quitting no matter what your age or how long you've smoked.

DRINK ALCOHOL IN MODERATION If you drink alcohol, keep it moderate — up to one drink a day for women of all ages.

SEEK REGULAR HEALTH CARE Checking in with your health care provider on a regular basis will ensure that you're getting the screening tests and preventive therapies that you need. In addition, taking an active role in your health can help you feel more competent and in control of your own body.

These habits are the same ones that stave off health problems in your younger years. You just might have to work twice as hard to maintain your health and vitality in the years after menopause.

Making peace with your changing body

Body image refers to your mental image or perception of your own physical appearance. It's formed by many factors and experiences, including your physical appearance, your weight, your values, your ethnic background, what you see in the media and what feedback you hear from others.

Menopause may also play a big role in your body image, just as puberty, pregnancy and other major life milestones altered how you felt in your own skin. Some women find the menopause transition to be liberating. Other women mourn the loss of their ability to have children and feel less desirable. Often, women experience complex, conflicting feelings of relief and sadness all at once.

During menopause, weight gain can also be a major concern and a major obstacle to a positive body image. For many women, menopause and aging affect metabolism, causing an uptick in weight without any real change in activity or diet. This feeling of a loss of control of your own weight can be frustrating, disheartening and inhibiting. You may find that you no longer feel comfortable in your favorite clothes — or without your clothes. In fact, many women say that weight gain gets in the way of feeling sexy and sexual.

Unfortunately, weight gain is unlikely to go away without significant effort. Even if you're able to maintain your premenopausal weight, you may carry it differently and feel thicker around your middle. So it's important to show yourself some compassion, even if you're not particularly fond of your new shape or size. In fact, studies show that having a positive body image and practicing self-compassion during menopause can actually result in fewer symptoms, including fewer hot flashes or night sweats that interfere with daily activities.

If you're struggling to be kind to yourself, try focusing on nonjudgmental presence and mindfulness. Look at your body and take note of the nooks, crannies and wrinkles. Look at them and describe exactly what you see without opinion or judgment. For example, instead of "I see flabby arms" (which is an opinion, not a fact), say "I see a larger patch of skin below my right arm. It feels soft and when I touch it, it moves from side to side" (this is a fact, not opinion). If judgment or the internal critic creeps in your mind (it surely will), let these negative thoughts go by, rather than letting them consume you or undermine your self-worth. These are just thoughts. You are not your thoughts. Let them float by like clouds in the sky and go back to the present moment. This is mindfulness. Keep practicing.

Although it's wise to focus on other things besides your looks as you age, a positive body image is still important. Having a positive view of your own body is essential for your confidence, satisfaction, sex life and self-esteem. Learning to take care of and love your body is crucial to your happiness.

Practical strategies for a better body image

If you don't like what you see in the mirror — or you've actually been avoiding a mirror for a while — it's time to make a change. Try new physical activities, and look at your body with a new perspective. These strategies can help:

GET MOVING! Exercise tends to make women feel better about their bodies, whether they lose weight or not. The type of exercise doesn't matter. Find something you like to do, and find a time to do it.

If you need extra motivation and accountability, sign up for an exercise class, work with a trainer, or make plans to meet a friend at the gym or park.

FOCUS ON PHYSICAL ACCOMPLISHMENTS Go rock climbing or paddle boarding. Take a cycling class or ballroom dancing class. Try footgolf or snorkeling with your kids or grandkids. Master a headstand or handstand. Jump off the diving board or the lakefront dock. Focus on all of the things that your body can do, not just how it looks.

If you're up for a challenge, sign up for a physical test that you've never tried before — such as a 5K walk or run, a dance class or even a short triathlon. Just make sure it's within your grasp, based on your abilities and physical health.

DON'T APOLOGIZE FOR YOUR BODY Whether you're wearing a swim-suit, workout clothes or a little black dress, there's no need to apologize for any blemishes in your appearance. Chances are, no one will notice any imperfections except you. There's no reason to call attention to them.

Did your mother ever tell you that if you can't say anything nice, you shouldn't say anything at all? Remember that when you talk about your own body. If you're not ready to be positive, at least stop making excuses and apologies. Pay attention to your body language, too. The way you move your body can seem like an apology even if you never say it out loud. Watch what others do when they're nervous, happy or sad. Use what you learn to control your body movements and send positive messages about how you feel about yourself.

DON'T CRITIQUE ANOTHER WOMAN'S CROW'S-FEET When you make snarky comments about how other women are aging poorly, you contrib-ute to the culture of unrealistic expectations about how women age. In addition, gossiping about other women affects your own body image. Your inner self can hear you.

Pay attention to how you talk about the appearance of other women — girlfriends, neighbors, co-workers, actresses and celebrities, aging female politicians, and other public figures. You may think that poking fun at other women — particularly public figures that you don't know personally — can make you feel better about your own looks. But, often, it's just the opposite. It's common to judge others the same way as you judge yourself.

WEAR THINGS THAT MAKE YOU FEEL GOOD ABOUT YOURSELF By the time you hit menopause, you're excused from following every fashion trend. Cultivate your own style, and wear things that make you feel good about yourself. If you feel good in jeans, make them your signature style. If you love dresses, don't bother saving them for fancy occasions. Play to your strengths. You know what they are.

Also, pay attention to accessories and other small luxuries that make you feel good, and wear them often. This might be a favorite perfume, a hand-me-down ring from your grandmother, a pair of lacy underwear or your perfectly worn-in cowboy boots.

DON'T DRAW YOUR BODY IMAGE FROM WHAT YOU SEE IN THE MEDIA Remember, these images are carefully produced by a huge team of experts who are trained to sell products or show celebrities in a positive light. The final result often bears little resemblance to reality. Don't be tempted to use these images as a yardstick to measure your own body.

ACCEPT AND VALUE YOUR GENES You probably inherited a lot of physical traits from your family. You might have your grandmother's hands or your favorite aunt's dimples. You probably have the same thick thighs and spider veins that these women had, too. Try to view these inherited traits as part of your pedigree and lineage. Embrace them just as you would embrace these beloved family members.

TAKE A GOOD LOOK AT YOUR OWN BODY Sometimes, the only way to move past a negative body image is to de-sensitize your feelings about your body. You can do this by really looking at your body in the mirror. Start by taking a hand mirror and looking at the different parts of your body. Begin with a part of your body that you're comfortable with — such as your hands. Look at your hands with curiosity. State the facts ("I see lines that extend from my wrist to knuckles that are raised and slightly darker than the rest of my hand"), not opinion ("I see veiny hands"). Really notice them. Then continue on to different parts of your body. Over time, you might be able to look in a larger mirror. This exercise may feel uncomfortable or awkward at first. That's OK. Keep practicing until you can experience your body factually and without judgment. Think about things you like about your body, such as your eyes, your smile, or that your arms allow you to paint or write.

THINK ABOUT YOUR PARTNER'S BODY Has your partner's body changed as you've aged together? Have these changes made your partner less lovable? What would you tell your partner if he or she was struggling to accept some of the changes that have occurred with age? Try listening to your own advice.

These strategies aren't meant to minimize the difficult task of loving your body as it ages. It's OK to grieve the loss of your younger, tauter self. Just remember that the stages of grief end with acceptance. So, if you find yourself stuck in the stage of anger or depression for a long time, it's a good idea to talk to your health care provider.

In fact, if you've struggled with your body image throughout your life, you may find that menopause triggers a recurrence of old feelings and doubts. You may benefit from counseling or other treatments to help with this transition. Support groups can also supply valuable information and help you connect with other women who share your experiences.

You are more than your body

The best way to fully embrace your postmenopausal self is a dichotomy. It's essential to foster a positive body image, even as your body changes in ways that you don't expect. Your goal is to accept your own figure, to stand tall in the mirror and to be comfortable having sex with the lights on. But it's equally important to recognize that you are much more than your body.

In your younger years, your physical attributes may actually have been your greatest assets. You may have been known for your great legs, your D-cup or your perfect bangs. That can be fun for a while, but of course, these features fade over time. And they're not much of a defining glory anyway.

In contrast, scientists have determined that personality generally doesn't change much after age 30. So your best inner qualities may stay with you forever and actually improve with age. Over time, your greatest asset might be your sharp wit, your knack for telling a great story or throwing a great party, your kindness to strangers, your stubborn streak, your passion for your work, your bravery during tough times, or your unwavering loyalty to friends. Isn't that a better legacy than enviable breasts?

As you work to embrace the woman in the mirror, remember to take a step back and think about all of the things that you can't see in your reflection. Focus on your whole self, not each fine line and sag. Some days, this may be more difficult than others. When that's the case, consider these final tips to help you gain a new perspective.

KEEP A LIST OF POSITIVE QUALITIES THAT HAVE NOTHING TO DO WITH YOUR APPEARANCE It's easy to be critical and focus on your flaws. Instead, focus on what makes you shine brightest. Write down a compliment or two for yourself and refer to it when you find yourself obsessing about your least favorite features. If you're not sure what to write, take note the next time a friend, neighbor or co-worker pays you a compliment. Or ask your partner to help you identify your greatest strengths.

SURROUND YOURSELF WITH PEOPLE WHO MAKE YOU FEEL GOOD ABOUT YOURSELF As a teenager, you probably had a few mean girls in your life — those spiteful, superficial girls who would smile nicely while making fun of your jeans. Unfortunately, there was some benefit to making nice with the mean girls, because they controlled the social pecking order and your chances of having somewhere to be on Saturday night.

At this stage in your life, there's no advantage to spending time with anyone who doesn't make you feel good about yourself. If you still have friends or family members in your life who constantly critique your choices or rain on your parade, it may be time for a breakup. At the very least, consider limiting your exposure to anyone who brings you down. Menopause is your license to close in your inner circle and to bask in the relationships that buoy you up.

ENGAGE IN HOBBIES OR ACTIVITIES THAT YOU ENJOY If you had a free afternoon with absolutely no obligations or limitations, how would you choose to spend it? On your bike? In your garden? At the theater? On a stool at the local wine bar with a girlfriend? With your nose in a new book? Baking bread? Playing the piano? There is no wrong answer here.

People who are involved in hobbies and leisure activities may be at a lower risk of some health problems. In addition, social activities and relaxing hobbies can help eliminate the stress and anxiety that keeps some women critical of their bodies. Make time for the passions and pursuits that you enjoy. Consider scheduling time for your hobbies on your calendar just as you would an important meeting, so they don't fall to the bottom of your priority list.

Also, consider sharing your hobbies or passions with your community in the form of volunteer work. If you love to cook or garden, you might volunteer at your local farmers market or soup kitchen. If you're a reader, you might relish a regular stint at the library. Older adults who participate in meaningful activities report feeling healthier and happier.

TALK TO OLDER WOMEN THAT YOU ADMIRE It's tough to feel bad about your aging body when you spend time with older women that you hold in high regard. Consider scheduling a semiregular coffee or lunch with one or two older woman whom you think highly of. It might be a favorite aunt, a long-time neighbor, a work mentor, or someone you've met through your hobbies or religious affiliation. You don't necessarily have to talk about the trials and tribulations of getting older, although you certainly could. Often, just spending time with older women role models will assure you that you're on the right path. If you don't have any women to fill this role in your life, consider reading biographies of accomplished women that you admire.

You may not be your own best cheerleader every day of the week. As your body changes, you're bound to have days when you don't feel very poised or confident. That's perfectly normal. Dust yourself off, be kind to yourself and keep going. With practice, you can develop a newfound confidence and richly deserved sense of empowerment as you embark on this next stage of your life.

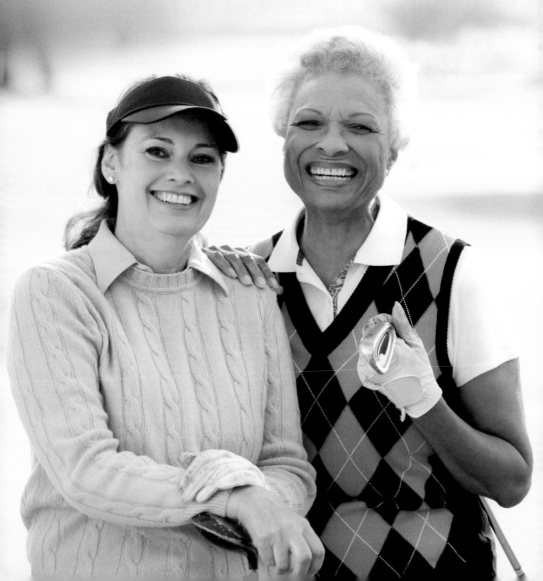

CHAPTER NINETEEN

Finding balance and happiness

Today, the average woman has more than one-third of her life ahead of her after menopause. That makes menopause a good time to take stock of your life and your priorities. Then, you can make changes to make the most of the coming years.

This new phase of life can be as relaxing and free or busy and fulfilling as you would like to make it. This is your chance to reset, reconnect, rearrange, reschedule and retune.

Of course, you can change your life's course at any time. But, for most people, meaningful change often happens on the heels of a clear defining moment — college graduation, marriage, parenthood, divorce, the death of a loved one, illness, a major job promotion, a cross-country move or retirement. Menopause can be in this category, and it often coincides with other major life changes as well — such as sending children off to college.

You only get a handful of these major milestones throughout your life, so it's wise to make them count. Take the time to pause and honor this transition in life. Then summon your inner strength and go for the life you really want. It's time.

Embrace your third act

By the time you reach the age of natural menopause, you've got decades of real living behind you. You've seen your fair share of places and presidencies and new technologies. You've had your heart broken. You've made mistakes and learned from them. You've fallen down and gotten back up and dusted yourself off. You've taken a leap. You've raised your babies — or helped raise someone else's babies. You've won awards, accolades, compliments and scars. You've forgiven and forgotten. You've learned what makes you tick and what brings you joy.

That doesn't mean it's all downhill from here. The third act is often the best. It's the climax of a chain of events, when something important is decided or made clear. As you write your own life story, use your time and energy wisely and embrace your third act. Build on all of the life experiences you have endured to date.

You'll need the right mindset to make this happen. Earlier in this book, you learned many strategies to make peace with your changing, aging body. Now, it's time to focus on your inner self, your values and your priorities for the future.

It all starts with your attitude, your perceptions and your beliefs about this new phase of life. These things are powerful forces, and they are within your control. So use them wisely.

If you feel down and negative about menopause and growing older, you have the power to reshape your attitude and build the life that you want. It will take some work. But you can do it. Here are some specific techniques to cultivate productive thinking and embrace the years ahead:

CHALLENGE YOUR NEGATIVE THOUGHTS Argue with them. Challenge their accuracy. Every time you challenge negative self-talk with facts, your negative thoughts lose their power. By changing your thoughts to be more accurate, you will eventually change the way you feel. You'll see that feelings of hopelessness, fear and anxiety can give way to feelings of power, courage, compassion and hope.

You can start by identifying any faulty thought patterns that get in your way and undermine your happiness. For example, maybe you tend to magnify the negative in a situation and filter out the positive. Say you're well-prepared and articulate for a work presentation and receive many compliments for a job well-done. But you stumble on the answer to one minor question from a challenging younger co-worker. That evening, you focus only on the misstep and forget about the accomplishment. Another common negative thought pattern is automatically jumping to conclusions and anticipating the worst in any situation. For example, you begin having hot flashes and immediately assume they're going to ruin your life.

In both of these situations, you can counter exaggerated negative self-talk ("My body is falling apart") with realistic thoughts ("I'm starting to have hot flashes, I should figure out self-care techniques or treatments that can help"). Find areas of your life that you often think negatively about, and think about ways to see them in a more positive, factual way.

FOCUS ON WHAT YOU CAN CONTROL Don't wallow in worry about the menopausal changes that you can't control. Instead, control your reaction to them. Reframe the situation as a challenge — not a catastrophe — and summon your inner strength to face change.

Take sleep problems, for example. You could keep yourself up all night worrying about sleep. Instead, control your reaction to the situation.

Problem-solve as much as possible. Buy cooler sheets and pajamas and get out your window fan. If you still have a bad night's sleep, reflect on what worked (the new pajamas) and what didn't (the fan was old and loud). Learn from your experiences (time to buy a new fan) and try again. Don't be discouraged if things don't always go your way. Shift your attention from helplessness and disappointment to planning mode. Commit to carrying out your plan before giving up or trying something else.

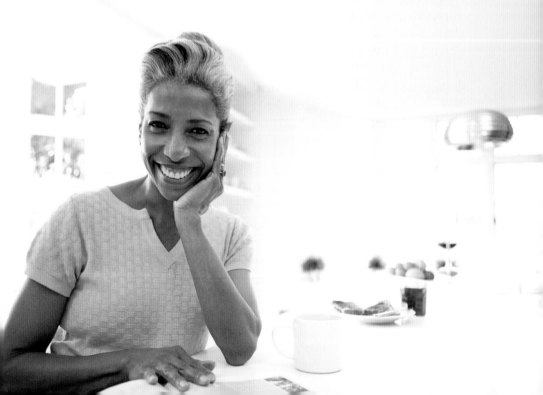

PRACTICE OPTIMISM That doesn't mean pretending menopause and all of its annoying symptoms are peachy when they're not. Nor does it mean ignoring some of the hard truths about this stage of life. Optimism is about looking for solutions and silver linings in times of hardship and stress.

Optimists experience disappointments just like everyone else, but they're able to view them as temporary events or roadblocks that must be gotten around. When optimists have a setback, they confine it to a specific event and don't allow it to contaminate every aspect of their lives. When optimists encounter a negative event, they don't take it as a personal insult or blame themselves for life's misfortune. Try out this view of the world and see if you can make it stick. It will help you live through your postmenopausal years with balance and joy.

Examine your values

Menopause is a time of change on many levels. Change is happening at the physical level, as your body stops producing estrogen — setting off a ripple effect of bothersome symptoms. At the same time, menopause can be a time of tumultuous life changes, when women are sandwiched between the needs of aging parents, growing adult children and midlife partners. Career success and responsibilities can be at an all-time high, too, leaving women stretched in all directions and feeling guilty that they're not doing everything right. As all of these demands converge, it can be tough to make yourself and your values a priority in your own life.

It's critical to use menopause as your opportunity to reflect and reassess your values and priorities. You only get 24 hours each day. How you spend that time is up to you. However, if you don't plan your time with clear intention, it's likely that others will fill up your time for you.

SKETCH OUT YOUR 'TIME PIE' Try the following exercise to record how your time is currently spent and what you would like to change. This exercise requires a sheet of paper, a pencil and 15 to 60 minutes of your undivided attention. Carve out a quiet time complete this exercise without interruptions. Make yourself a cup of tea or pour yourself a glass of wine and plan to take your time with this exercise.

Draw a circle on a sheet of paper. Then divide it up into segments that represent the number of hours you spend for various activities on a typical day, adding up to 24 hours. Fill in the number of hours you spend for:

- Sleep
- Work
- Chores
- Commute
- Caregiving
- Errands
- Family time
- Significant other relationship
- Technology and device use
- Exercise
- Fun

Label each slice of the pie with the activity and the number of typical hours you spend doing it each day. Be as accurate as possible.

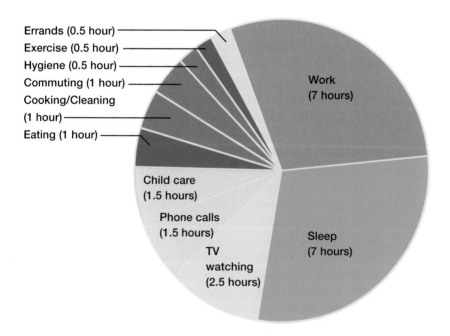

Now, take a good look at the pie you've sketched. Do the results surprise you? Is there a slice that's much bigger or smaller than you would have thought? Is there a slice that's much bigger or smaller than you would like?

To help, give some thought to the following questions. Pondering these questions will help you identify what experiences and values are most important to you:

▶ What are your most important relationships?
▶ Where have you found comfort?
▶ What do you most value in your life?
▶ Which people give you a sense of community?
▶ What inspires you and gives you hope?
▶ What brings you joy?
▶ What are your three most memorable experiences?
▶ What are your proudest achievements?

How does your pie compare to your answers to the questions above? Are the things that bring you joy part of your pie? Are the things you value most in your life part of your pie? How many things appear both on your pie and in the answers to the questions above? Two? Three? Five?

If your typical day and your values are divergent, create one more pie that represents your ideal day. In your ideal world, how would you devote your time and energy? How would you like to spend your day?

Chances are, your typical day and your ideal day are not the same. That's a natural consequence of being an adult and having responsibilities and commitments. However, there should be some overlap and synergy. When you have little time to spend on the things that really matter to you, it can be a source of stress that keeps you from being your best self.

Think about lifestyle changes you can make so that your typical pie and your ideal pie are a little closer. You probably can't quit your job to spend more time with the people you love. But you may be able to slim down the work slice of your pie by cutting back on nighttime work emails or weekend trips to the office in order to find more time for your family. Or perhaps you could outsource some errands or change the amount of time you're spending in front of the TV to make room for the things that bring you joy. Aligning your daily choices with your values can bring meaning and purpose to your days. If you have neglected certain joys for years, relegating them to your lowest priority, now is your time to turn it around.

Think about one or two specific changes that you would like to make. Develop a plan to make these changes, and take action. Consider saving your drawings and repeating this exercise in a month or two to see your progress. It will take time and effort to shift the size of your slices. Be patient with yourself. Monitor how your plan is working and make adjustments as you go.

KNOW YOUR 'BIG ROCKS' Of course, there are many ways to rethink your priorities. If the time pie exercise doesn't resonate with you, try reflecting on the following story. This story has been told for years in many different versions. It provides another way to visualize your values:

One day, a college professor put a mason jar on the table in front of his students. Then he produced a bucket of big rocks and began placing them into the jar. When the jar was filled to the top and no more rocks would fit inside, he asked the students, "Is the jar full?" The students said "yes."

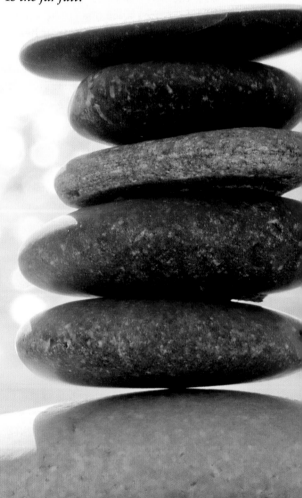

But the professor proved them wrong by unveiling a bucket of pebbles and adding them to the jar. The professor was able to fit a lot of pebbles around all of the big rocks. "Is the jar full now?" he asked. By this time, the students were a bit wiser and they shook their heads "no."

This was the correct response, as the professor then produced a bucket of sand and poured sand around all of the big rocks and small pebbles. "Now is it full?" he asked. "Probably not," the class said. And they were correct. The professor took out a pitcher of water and filled the jar to the brim.

"Now the jar is really full," the professor declared. *"What is the point of this demonstration?"*

One student raised his hand and guessed that the point was, no matter how full your schedule is, you can always accomplish more. But, in fact, that was not the point the professor was trying to make. His intention was to show how important it is to start with the big rocks. "If you put the water, sand and pebbles in the jar before the big rocks," he told the students, *"you would never accommodate the big rocks."*

How wise. Menopause is an opportunity to identify your big rocks and build your life around your big rocks. You won't have time to adjust the big rocks again, once you pour in the sand and the pebbles. So it's important to choose your big rocks carefully and anchor them firmly.

Ask yourself: What are your big rocks? Your family? Your faith? Your job? A hobby you're passionate about, such as biking or playing the piano? A cause that's near and dear to your heart?

You have a lot of responsibilities, but only some are big rocks. The rest are pebbles and sand. Know the difference. There is not enough time in the day to get everything done every day. But you can mitigate a lot of stress in your life if you focus on the big rocks and do the things that really matter to you.

Learning to say no

As noted earlier in this chapter, the years surrounding menopause are often very busy years in women's lives, full of competing priorities. Some of your frenzy may be the result of very good things that occur at this stage of life — such as planning a child's wedding, taking on a leadership role at work or accepting a position on the board of a favorite charity. Other responsibilities are not so pleasant — such as caring for aging parents, helping a friend through a divorce, or worrying about financing your retirement or children's college educations. All of these stressors — good and bad — can take a toll. You will only find balance and happiness when you protect your time and set limits, according to the values and "big rocks" you have identified.

WHEN TO SAY NO At this time in life, you may receive a lot of requests for your hard-earned wisdom and expertise. This can be flattering. Sometimes it's tough to determine which activities deserve your time and attention. Use these strategies to evaluate obligations — and opportunities — that come your way.

Focus on what matters most Remember your big rocks. When an opportunity or commitment comes your way, think about whether it is a big rock that's worthy of your time and attention. Is the new commitment important to you? Or is it just another item on your to-do list?

Assess the time commitment Is the new activity you're considering a short- or long-term commitment? Even if a volunteer commitment passes the "big rock" test, it's important to remember that signing up for a single Saturday event will take far less time than heading up the whole fundraising committee. Be realistic about what you can handle. Don't overcommit yourself at home, work, church or in your community.

Let go of guilt Don't agree to a request you would rather decline out of guilt or obligation. Saying no is not a sign of rudeness. There are times when you have to say no, even to people you love. If your parents or in-laws want to get together for an impromptu dinner when you've already scheduled a quiet evening at home with your partner, it's OK to decline their offer. Set realistic goals for what you can — and want — to accomplish.

Sleep on it Stop saying yes to requests on the spot. When someone asks you to do something, get in the habit of saying that you're flattered and you'll respond with a firm answer in the next day or so. Or ask them to send you an email with this request. If they do send you an email (often they won't!), this buys you time to mull over a new opportunity and decide if it really fits into your current commitments and priorities. You may find that your excitement for a new opportunity waxes or wanes overnight. This is a good indicator of whether you should sign on.

HOW TO SAY NO Don't be afraid to say no. Remember that sometimes you have to say no" in order to say yes to things that matter most. Still, it can be difficult to disappoint people who want your help and time. Sometimes the people who request your assistance are in a vulnerable spot; handle your response tenderly.

Be clear about saying no Be careful not to use wimpy substitute phrases such as "I'm not sure" or "I don't think I can." These can be interpreted to mean that you might say yes later.

Practice full disclosure Don't make up reasons to get out of an obligation. The truth is always the best way to turn someone down.

Let them down gently It can be tough to turn down good causes that land at your door. Compliment the person or group's effort while saying that you're unable to commit at this time. A respectful approach shows that you're just turning down a commitment, not snubbing the group's mission or accomplishments.

Cushion your response to a loved one Try using the "sandwiched no": yes-no-yes. Begin with initial, honest enthusiasm ("I would love to"); follow with a polite no that includes a proper explanation ("I have too much going on"); and finish with a second-best option that partially compensates for your no ("How about next Monday?"). Your no then becomes a "half-yes," which is easier to swallow.

Finally, soften your no with something else that shows you care. For example, say your partner asks you to meet for lunch on a workday, but you need to work through your lunch hour. If you can't go to lunch, surprise your partner with a card or bring home a box of chocolates that he or she loves. It'll prevent an unpleasant experience from becoming a black hole.

Saying no won't be easy if you're used to saying yes all the time. But it will get easier over time. Remind yourself that learning to say no is an important way to shine in your postmenopausal years.

Caring for yourself

You may wonder why it's necessary to redefine your priorities and learn to say no to some of the obligations and opportunities that come your way. Why can't you just continue on the same old track that you've been plodding down for decades? The big reason is you!

As you navigate the transition to menopause, it's critical to reclaim your rightful place on your own list of priorities. The physical symptoms of menopause and aging are exacerbated when you don't take care of yourself. In addition, medical illnesses and changes in your overall health can occur at this time if you don't take precautions to preserve or improve your health.

Where do you fall on your own priority list? In your 30s and 40s, you may have relegated yourself to a mere sliver of your time pie, as you focused your attention on building a nest, a family and a career. While common, this tactic won't serve you well as you age. A healthy balance between work, caring for others and taking care of yourself is important to your well-being. It's time to find your voice and be an advocate for your own wants and needs.

Earlier in this book, you learned about many lifestyle changes that can protect or improve your health at this time of life. As you know by now, the short list includes moving more, eating well, quitting smoking, limiting alcohol, establishing a healthy sleep routine and keeping up on regular appointments with your health care provider. Beyond these important lifestyle habits, there are other things you can do to care for your body and spirit during this stage of life:

TAKE A RESPITE FROM CAREGIVING If you are a caregiver for aging parents, give yourself a break. Many women who are actively caring for older adults don't identify as a "caregiver." Recognizing this role and the emotional and physical demands involved with caregiving can help you seek out support.

Let those in your care be as independent as possible. It's tempting to accompany Mom and Dad to every doctor's appointment and to be at their beck and call for household chores. But it's important to differentiate between the things your parents can handle on their own and the tasks they need you for. This distinction is good for both of you.

In addition, accept help from others. If siblings, neighbors or family friends offer to assist, say yes. Be prepared with a list of specific ways that others can help, such as taking your parents to the grocery store or mowing their lawn. Don't be too proud to accept help for yourself as well. Caring for aging parents is a big job. If friends know you're spending a lot of time in this role and offer to bring you a meal, graciously accept it. Allowing others to help you actually helps your parents.

In addition, be sure to take advantage of resources and tools in your community that can help you help your loved one. Many communities have classes and services, such as transportation and meal delivery, that could ease your load. Your health care provider, your parent's provider or a support group for caregivers can help you find resources and solve common caregiving problems.

Many women who are caring for aging parents are also caring for teenagers or young adults and are divided in their responsibilities. If you're in this situation, you probably want to be a supermom and a superdaughter and a superworking woman and a superwife. But your self-care can suffer if you try to hold yourself to superstandards. Try to let go of guilt and be realistic about what you can accomplish. Don't compromise your sleep, your time for exercise or your healthy-eating habits trying to do it all. Remember, if you don't take care of yourself, you won't be able to care for those who need you.

TAKE TIME TO DO SOMETHING YOU WANT TO DO This was discussed in the previous chapter, but it's worth repeating. Too often, women don't take time to do the things they really want to do until they've finished all of their responsibilities and commitments to others. Doing things in this order leaves too little — sometimes zero — time for the things you really want to do.

Instead of saving your passions and hobbies for that rare free moment, schedule them into your day. Book a block of time for gardening. Schedule a meeting with your favorite book and your favorite sunny spot. Get up early and make a trail run or yoga class the first thing you do, rather than the last. Time spent doing the things you love is not wasted time. It allows you to recharge and attend to your responsibilities with new energy and vigor.

PAMPER YOURSELF Treat yourself to a massage, manicure or bubble bath. Escape to a local concert or theater show. Meet your best friend for a cup of tea or coffee. Buy a new novel or a pair of earrings you've been coveting. Enjoy an alfresco glass of champagne with your partner, and toast your fabulous self. Shower yourself with something special — it doesn't have to be expensive or fancy.

TAKE CARE OF YOUR SPIRIT This is different for everyone. For some, it takes the form of religious observance, prayer, meditation or a belief in a higher power. For others, it is found in nature, music, art or a secular community. Staying connected to your inner spirit and the lives of those around you can enhance your quality of life, both mentally and physically. Your personal concept of spirituality may change with your age and life experiences, but it always forms the basis of your well-being, helps you cope with stressors large and small, and affirms your purpose in life.

STAY CURIOUS Stretch yourself by trying new things as you age. Take a class at your local art or pottery studio. Or look into adult or continuing education classes in your area. You've always wanted to try a Pilates, creative writing or gourmet pasta-making class, right? Traveling is another way to expand your horizons and gain new perspective. If you can't book a trip to a far-flung destination right now, at least consider a reservation at the new ethnic restaurant in your hometown.

LAUGH Loud. And often. It really is the best medicine. Be silly with your grandkids, nieces or nephews. Spend time with girlfriends who keep you giggling. Or rent a movie that appeals to your sense of humor.

Try to let go of any guilt that you feel when you take time for yourself. It's not selfish or lazy to prioritize a bubble bath or an afternoon of painting. It's self-assertive. Think of these activities as part of your doctor's orders to take care of yourself. If you find that you can't let go of the guilt, practice mindfulness. Notice the guilt, be curious about it and then redirect your attention back to the present moment (the paint on your canvas or the warmth of the bubble bath).

Nourish your relationship

At this stage in life, another winning way to take care of yourself is to take care of your relationship with your partner. You will need your partner's love and support as you grow old together, but your relationship can take a hit at this time if you don't pay special attention to it. As you learned in Chapter 7, sexual problems and relationship issues are common during menopause. You may need to work to add spice to and cultivate novelty in your relationship.

FIND NOVELTY Novelty is your appreciation of uniqueness. Something novel is interesting, original, contrasting, unique, exclusive or beyond usual expectations. Novelty is in the eyes of the beholder. For example, the technology in an airplane cockpit is novel for most people, but not for a pilot; a video of a beating heart is novel for the pilot, but not for a cardiologist.

How can you keep your relationship fresh each day — especially if you've been together for decades? Try this exercise: Imagine being away alone on a 10-day business trip. When you come home, are you more likely to meet your partner with a more loving presence, at least for the first 15 minutes?

Now, think about how you feel about your partner on a regular basis. When you see your loved ones every day, they become familiar, even bordering on boring. When you haven't seen them for 10 days, your system perceives one attribute that draws the mind's attention — novelty.

So here is your challenge: Can you greet your partner at the end of each day as if you're seeing him or her for the first time after 10 days? This develops a fresh relationship each time you meet. Can you give your partner at least the same attention that you bestow on your favorite gadget or a friend who you haven't seen for a long time? Can you challenge yourself to celebrate a little when you meet your loved ones at the end of the day?

Bring your nonjudgmental presence. Show your excitement at being together. Try not to fold laundry or scan through email during the first 15 minutes of reconnecting. Instead, do your best to give your partner your undivided attention. Try to fall in love with a new partner every day, in the same person.

This won't always be easy. Sometimes, when you see your partner at the end of a long day, the timing will be inconvenient. You will be in the midst of other tasks — thinking about a work problem, trying to get dinner

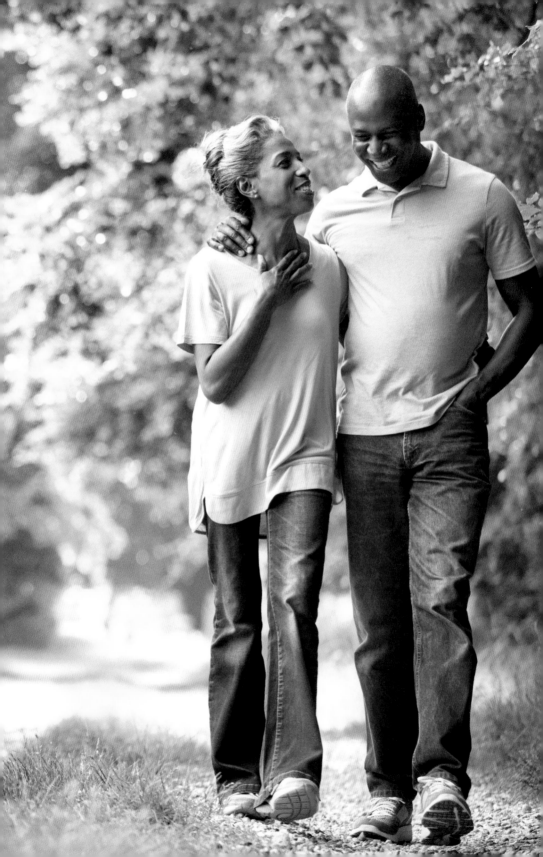

started, adding things to your mental to-do list, or simply enjoying a moment of peace and quiet. All of these things are important. However, challenge yourself to make a conscious decision to abandon them for just 15 minutes to be present for your partner. Take 15 minutes to talk about your day, flirt and catch up. You may be amazed at the difference that these 15 minutes can make in your relationship.

How to help your partner help you

If menopause caught you off guard, you're not alone. The range of changes that can occur as estrogen gradually declines can be surprising.

Now, think about your partner. If you were caught off guard by the changes that are occurring in your body, your partner may be downright baffled or befuddled.

Let's be honest. Loving a woman in menopause isn't always easy. It can be confusing or disorienting when the person you love suddenly changes dramatically in ways that you weren't expecting — even if the changes are a normal part of the aging process.

If you're more moody, overheated, exhausted, anxious, dejected or private than you've ever been before, your partner may not know what to do. Some men actually worry that their partner is having an affair during menopause, because emotions and sexual appetites can change so substantially and abruptly.

You may need to schedule an estrogen 101 talk with your partner. Briefly remind your partner how estrogen works in the body (refer back to Chapters 1 and 3 if you need to), and explain the changes that you're feeling. Be honest. Let your partner know that you may need a little extra support, patience and kindness as you work your way through the challenges of menopause. Research shows that a supportive, loving partner can actually help reduce menopausal stress and ease symptoms.

Talk to your partner about the symptoms that you're experiencing and give specific examples of changes in your home and relationship that might help. For example, let your partner know if you need to cool down your bedroom for a good night's sleep. Discuss how more lubrication or a vibrator may help during sex. Be honest if weight gain is bothering you and you want to shift your family schedule to attend a new class at the gym.

If open, honest communication isn't a hallmark of your relationship, you may be in for some tough talks. Consider working with a counselor to discover ways to communicate better and rekindle your relationship.

PRACTICE POSITIVITY In addition, keep a close eye on your positivity-negativity (P-N) ratio, a concept used by psychology professor and marriage researcher John Gottman. Positivity refers to encouraging positive feedback you provide to others, while negativity represents negative feedback. The higher your P-N ratio, the more you thrive in a relationship. Gottman's research suggests that you need five instances of positive feedback to neutralize one instance of negative feedback. He found that most teams with excellent dynamics, including successful marriages, have a high P-N ratio (typically greater than 5), while marriages at risk of divorce have a low ratio (often less than 1).

Ask yourself: How many consistent, fresh deposits have you made into your partner's positivity account lately? Think back to yesterday. Did you compliment your partner's new shirt? Did you kiss your partner before you left for work or went to sleep? Did you pick up your partner's dry-cleaning or buy a favorite treat at the grocery store? Did you eat dinner together? Every small act of kindness, every soothing word and every expression of approval creates a deposit. The little things that you do make a profound difference. Showing understanding, meeting expectations, making good on promises, sincerely apologizing — all enhance the P-N ratio.

Share this idea with your partner, and work together to keep the positivity flowing at your home and boost your ratio. Yes, there are times where honest criticism is appropriate. But you really can't have too much positivity. Nobody ever complains about being overappreciated. Intentionally upping your positive instances and noting your negative instances will allow you to strengthen your connections and energy. It won't be easy every day, but it's worth a sincere try.

Also, remember that not everyone is good with words. Some people are kind with words. Others are kind with deeds. Only a rare few are kind with both. If your partner isn't good with words, take note of his or her deeds — such as making you a cup of coffee, snuggling up next to you on the couch, filling up the gas in your car, sitting in the kitchen while you cook or holding your hand. Recognize these deeds for what they are — acts of praise and love for you. These actions are just as powerful as a verbal compliment or profession of love.

INVEST YOUR TIME Finally, invest in quality time with your partner. If you've been in your relationship for a long time, you may feel as if you've grown distant from your partner, even if you're regularly in the same room. This is common. Your time together may be stuffed with chores and obligations — keeping the house in order and entertaining business clients, for example. But that's all you have time for. You're committed to each other, but you're too busy to spend real quality time together.

How can you change that? Could you schedule a date night once a week? Could you buy season tickets to a concert series or theater series so that you have a series of evenings out planned? Could you take a class together, such as a spinning class or a wine-tasting class? Could you commit to setting aside just 10 or 20 minutes every day to talk or go for a walk or do something enjoyable together, such as gardening, playing cards or reading the newspaper?

You only get so much time with the people you love. When you spend this time wisely, you will make deeper connections and foster intimacy. And your life will be better for it.

Moving forward with the new you

Today is your day. Tomorrow is your day. And the next day is your day, too. Midlife is a time of opportunity and promise.

Yes, it's a time of change — physical changes, emotional ups and downs, and social adjustments. But it's also a time to take the reins and make changes of your own. The choices you make now can help you transform your health, your relationship and your life for decades to come. So make them strong choices.

Set your expectations high. Your expectations are a powerful thing. Use them to carve out the life you really want.

It's never too late to turn out some of your best work. Many women before you have blazed a trail of achievements after age 50:

▶ Julia Child didn't enroll in cooking school until she was almost 40 and didn't launch her popular TV show until she was 50.

▶ Laura Ingalls Wilder published the first *Little House* book when she was 65 and completed the last book when she was 76.

▶ Juliette Gordon Low founded the Girl Scouts at age 52.

▶ Mother Teresa received the Nobel Peace Prize in 1979 at age 69.

- After withdrawing from artistic life for a couple of years, artist Georgia O'Keefe returned to painting and sculpting at the age of 86 and went on to receive the National Medal of Arts.

- At the age of 88, actress Betty White became the oldest person to guest-host "Saturday Night Live." She earned glowing reviews and an Emmy Award for her appearance.

- Sandra Day O'Connor took her seat on the Supreme Court at the age of 51, and she retired at the age of 76.

What triumphs or crowning accomplishments might you achieve in your third act of life? What dreams can you dream for yourself? Expand your horizons, enjoy yourself and make your third act worthy of a standing ovation.

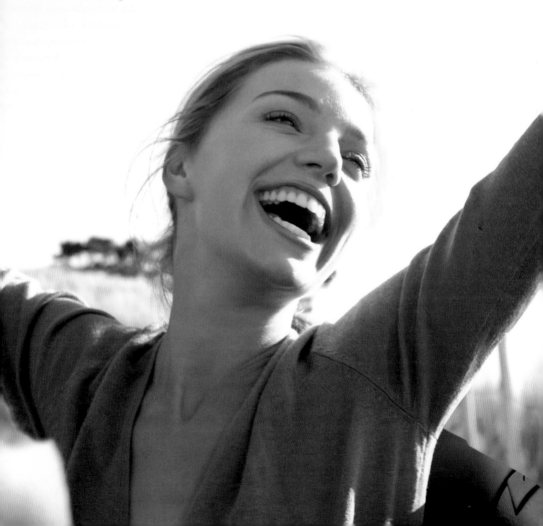

INDEX

dry skin, 57
dual energy X-ray absorptiometry (DXA), 222–223
dyspareunia. *See* sexual pain

E

ear protection, 268–269
Early Versus Late Intervention Trial with Estradiol (ELITE), 255
embryo cryopreservation, 46–47
emotional support, 45
employment/income changes, 80
endometrial hyperplasia, 141–142
energy balance, 150–152
energy therapies, 185
erectile dysfunction, 123
estradiol, 43
estriol, 167
estrogen
conjugated, 167
defined, 26, 167
fluctuation in levels of, 27, 28–29
low levels of, 41–42
in maintaining bone density, 231
as medication, 122–123
protective effects on neurons, 251–252
thermoneutral zone and, 71
estrogen therapy (ET), 167
estrogen-progestogen therapy (EPT), 167
estrone, 167
evening primrose oil, 191–192
excess body weight, impacts of, 147
exercise
aerobic activities, 247
amount needed, 156–158
in bone loss prevention, 226–227
brain benefits of, 258–260
daily activities as, 247
getting, 298
goals, 15
in heart-healthy lifestyle, 246–247
improvements gained by, 14–15
at menopause, 155–158
multiple benefits of, 157
power of, 155–156
in reducing breast cancer risk, 216
restless legs and, 107
sleep and, 17, 100
sleep apnea and, 105
strength training, 156, 227
stress-reducing, 90

in treating depression, 84
weight management and, 151, 155–158
weight-bearing, 227
eye changes
dry eyes, 53, 265–267
everyday care, 267
hormone therapy and, 173
sex hormones and, 52
types of, 52–53
eye examinations, 267, 284–285
eye health, 19

F

facial hair, 51–52
falls, preventing, 228
family history
breast cancer risk and, 210
heart disease and, 237–239
premature menopause and, 41
urinary incontinence and, 132
fat distribution, 148–149
female reproductive system, 129–130
fertility preservation, 46
fiber, 153
fish oil, 196
fitness, focus on, 14–15
flossing, 270
follicle-stimulating hormone (FSH)
defined, 26
evaluating levels of, 43
Fracture Risk Assessment Tool (FRAX) calculator, 221–222
freezing eggs, 47
freezing embryos, 46–47
fruits and vegetables, 245, 267, 268

G

genetic disorders, 40
genetic screening, 214
genitourinary syndrome of menopause (GSM), 59–60, 113
gingivitis, 55
ginkgo, 194–195
ginseng, 192, 195
gratitude
aging with, 296–298
defined, 296
journal, 296
practice of, 89
starting day with, 296
guilt, letting go of, 314
gum infections, 55

H

hair
  damage, avoiding, 262–263
  thinning, solutions for, 263–264
  unwanted, 264–265
hair changes, 51, 173, 262–265
hair loss, 51
headaches, 276
health
  addressing, 41–42
  bone, 41
  cardiovascular, 41
  exercise and, 14
  mood and, 79
  sexual, 42
  sleep and, 97
  stress impact on, 20
health care, seeking, 299
health care provider
  in premature menopause, 42–43
  sharing information with, 13
healthy diet
  balanced approach, 152
  fiber focus, 153
  foundations of, 152–155
  heart, 244–246
  portion size, 154
  in weight management, 15, 151,
    152–154
  See also diet
healthy weight
  defined, 146
  determining, 147–150
  exercise and, 156
  eye care and, 267
  in heart-healthy lifestyle, 247
  maintaining, 298
  Mayo Clinic Healthy Weight
    Pyramid, 153
  in reducing breast cancer risk, 215
hearing changes, 53–54, 267–269
hearing test, 285
Heart and Estrogen-Progestin Replace-
    ment Study (HERS), 254
heart disease
  aspirin and, 240–241
  blood pressure and, 237
  diabetes and, 237–239
  diagnosing in women, 240
  family history and, 239
  high cholesterol and, 234–237
  hormone therapy and prevention
    of, 243

menopause and, 232–233
risks of, 234–239
signs and symptoms in women, 236
heart-healthy diet, 244–246
heart-healthy lifestyle
  exercise, 246–247
  healthy diet, 244–246
  healthy weight, 247
  tobacco avoidance, 243–244
heart problems more common in
    women, 235
heart protection strategies, 239–242
  aspirin, 240–241
  statins, 241–242
hepatitis C testing, 286
hobbies/activities, 304
hormones
  brain and, 250–255
  changes during lifetime, 25–28
  depression and, 80–81
  fluctuating levels, 27
  key, list of, 26
  levels, testing, 43
  skin and, 55–56
  sleep and, 96
  vagina and vulva and, 58–59
  See also specific hormones
hormone therapy, 164–179
  alternative preparations, 174–177
  basic principles of, 165
  benefits of, 42–43, 165
  bioidentical custom-compound
    hormones, 176–177
  brain and, 254
  breakthrough bleeding risk, 171
  breast cancer risk and, 216
  defined, 166
  delivery methods, 169–170
  for depression, 85
  dosage, 171
  dosing schedule, 170–171
  duration, 171–174
  effectiveness, 165
  expert opinion of, 165
  follow-up care, 178
  headaches and, 276
  health considerations, 172–173
  healthy lifestyle choices with, 179
  historical background, 166–167
  in maintaining bone density, 231
  in premature menopause, 30,
    42–44, 177
  preparations, 170–171

restless legs syndrome, 106–107
rosacea, 57

S

MAYO CLINIC, a not-for-profit institution, recognizes a moral responsibility to provide whole-person care to everyone who needs healing. It is dedicated to providing comprehensive diagnosis and care in every medical specialty. With this depth of expertise, Mayo Clinic occupies a unique position as a resource to help people lead healthier lives. Mayo Clinic has published reliable health information for millions of consumers worldwide since 1983. Revenues support Mayo Clinic programs, including medical education and research.

ABOUT THE MAYO CLINIC WOMEN'S HEALTH CLINIC

The multidisciplinary Mayo Clinic Women's Health Clinic team includes specialists in internal medicine, endocrinology, geriatrics, gynecology, psychology, dermatology and physical therapy, who partner to provide collaborative, innovative, evidence-based care for women. Services provided by the Women's Health Clinic team are tailored to meet the unique needs of each woman, helping her optimize her overall health and well-being.

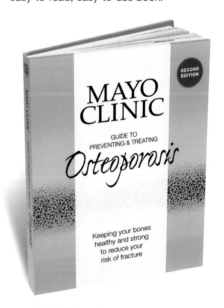